MW00893724

30-MINUTE MEDITERRANEAN DIET COOKBOOK FOR BEGINNERS

120 Quick and Easy Recipes
for Healthy Weight Loss and Vibrant Living

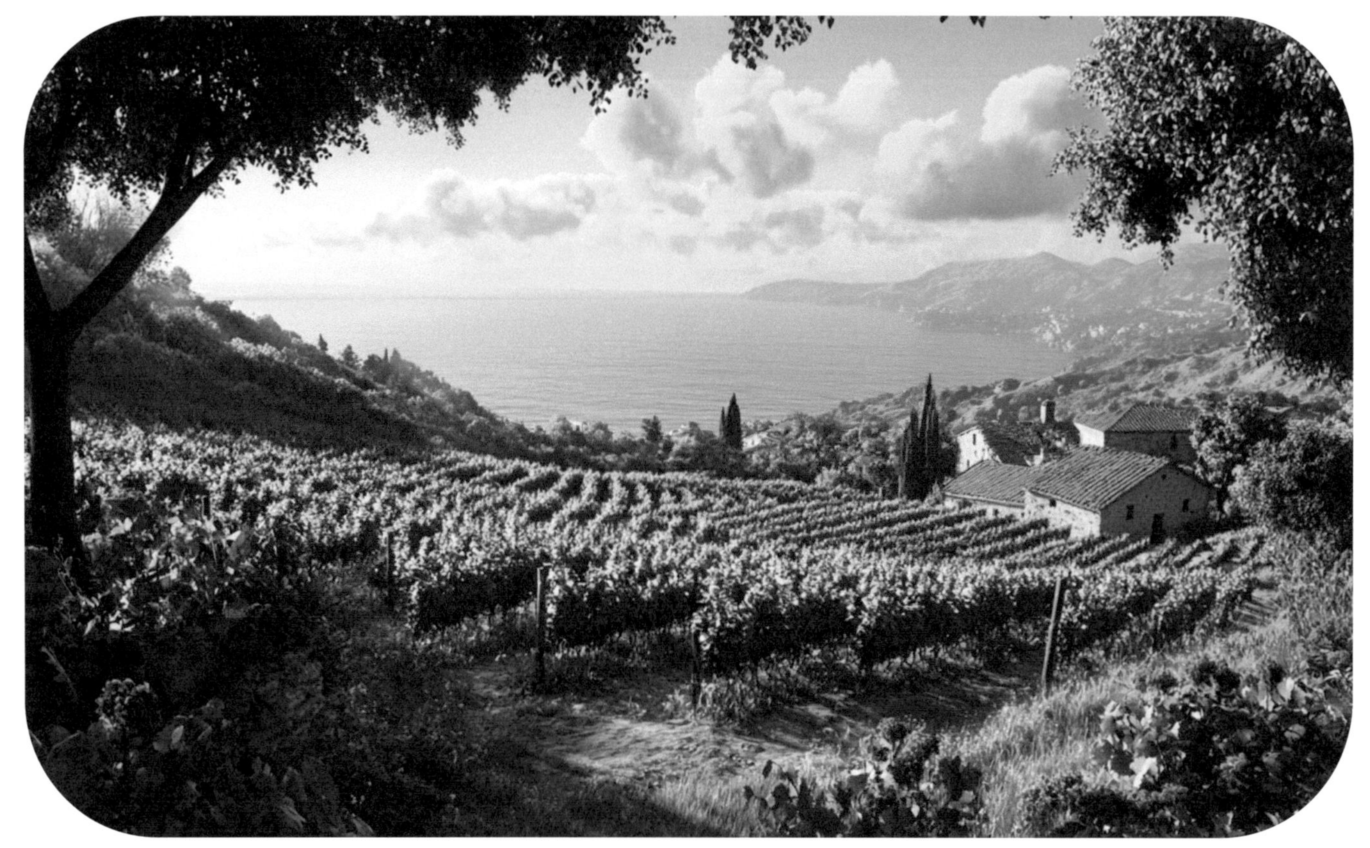

TABLE of CONTENTS

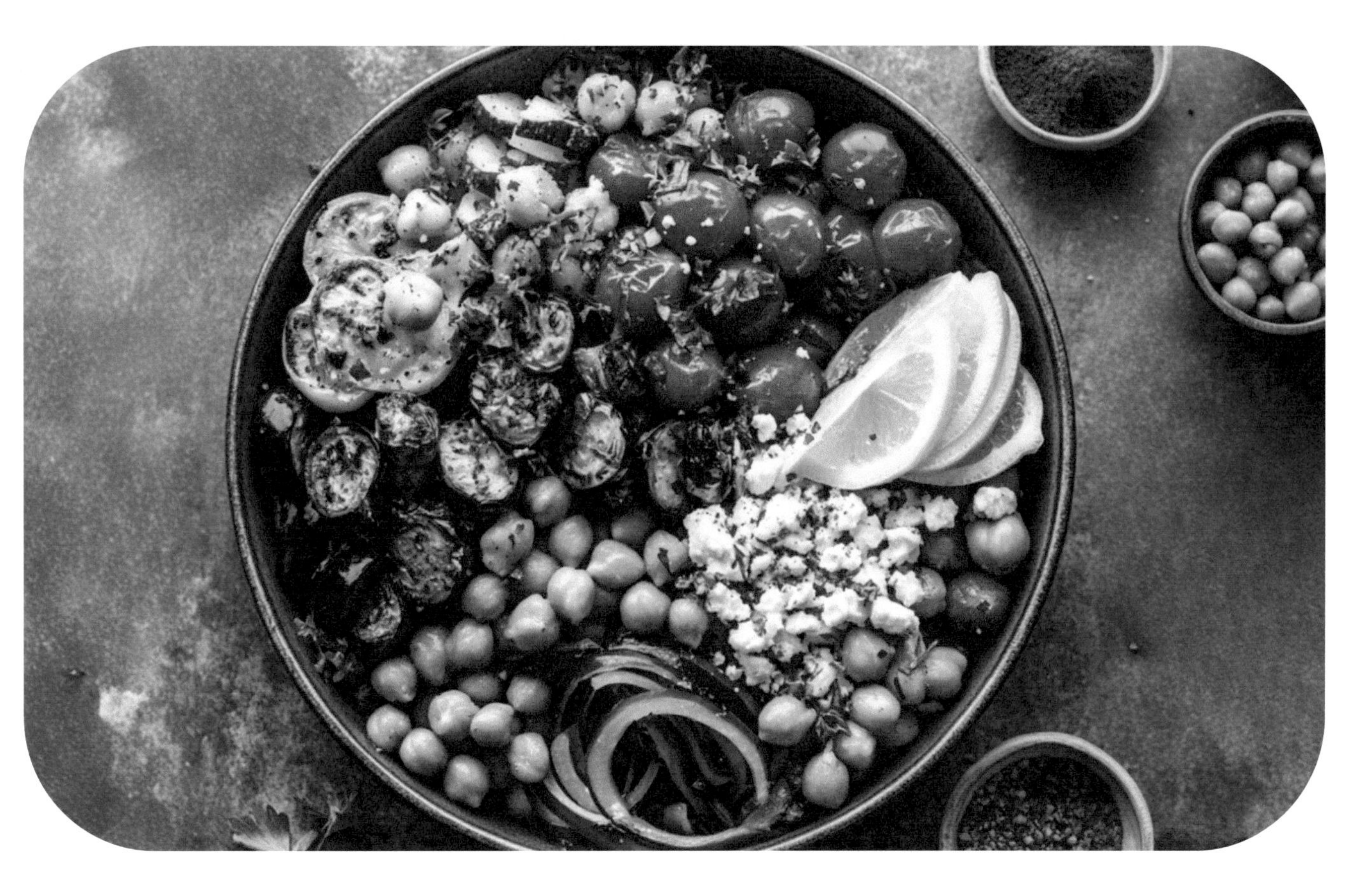

INTRODUCTION

Welcome to the **"30-Minute Mediterranean Diet Cookbook for Beginners"**—your guide to the delicious flavors, simplicity, and health benefits of the Mediterranean lifestyle. More than just a diet, it's a way of life rooted in balance, nourishment, and the joy of sharing meals with loved ones. Whether you're new to the Mediterranean diet or looking for quick, healthy meals, this cookbook is here to make every dish a flavorful and effortless experience. With a focus on fresh, wholesome ingredients, this book transforms everyday cooking into a journey of health, satisfaction, and discovery.

Inside, you'll find easy recipes crafted with wholesome ingredients and clear, beginner-friendly instructions, proving that healthy cooking doesn't have to be complicated. From vibrant breakfasts to satisfying dinners, every recipe is ready in 30 minutes or less—perfect for busy lifestyles. Whether you're cooking for one, two, or the whole family, these dishes are designed to fit seamlessly into your day while delivering bold flavors and maximum nourishment.

Discover the heart of Mediterranean cooking, where fresh vegetables, whole grains, healthy fats, and lean proteins come together in nourishing and satisfying meals. With flexible, creative recipes, you'll enjoy the freedom to adapt dishes to your taste while embracing the joy of cooking at home. From the tangy zest of lemons to the richness of olive oil and the boldness of fresh herbs, each recipe reflects the vibrant traditions of Mediterranean cuisine.

This cookbook makes healthy eating simple, enjoyable, and accessible. It empowers you to embrace a lifestyle that supports both physical and mental well-being while celebrating the pleasure of delicious food. Let it inspire you to create quick, wholesome meals that bring both flavor and well-being to your table.

Welcome to a healthier, more delicious way of life—one that's ready in just 30 minutes!

Welcome to 30-Minute Mediterranean Cooking

Welcome to the vibrant world of Mediterranean cooking—a timeless tradition rooted in fresh, seasonal ingredients and a rich cultural heritage. Spanning the coasts of Greece, Italy, Spain, and North Africa, this style of cooking celebrates the simplicity of wholesome foods like olive oil, grains, vegetables, and seafood. Meals are designed to be shared, creating a sense of connection and joy around the table.

The Mediterranean diet is more than just food—it's a way of life that values balance, flavor, and mindfulness. By combining fresh produce, lean proteins, and healthy fats with simple yet bold flavors, it offers a nourishing and delicious approach to eating. This tradition also encourages savoring each meal and embracing the pleasure of cooking and sharing food.

Renowned for its health benefits, including improved heart health and reduced inflammation, the Mediterranean diet is as good for your body as it is for your taste buds. In this book, you'll learn how to bring the vibrant flavors and healthful benefits of Mediterranean cooking into your busy life, creating satisfying meals in just 30 minutes or less.

The Mediterranean Diet: A Journey to Better Health

The Mediterranean diet isn't just a passing trend—it's a lifestyle deeply rooted in centuries of tradition and wisdom. Originating from the coastal regions of Greece, Italy, Spain, and North Africa, this approach to eating has been celebrated for its incredible health benefits and delicious flavors. It focuses on fresh vegetables, whole grains, lean proteins, and healthy fats, creating meals that are both nutritious and satisfying.

This diet has been extensively studied and shown to improve heart health, enhance brain function, reduce inflammation, and promote longevity. But it's more than just about health—it's a way of life that celebrates balance, sustainability, and the joy of eating mindfully. By adopting this lifestyle, you're not only nourishing your body but also embracing a tradition of enjoying food that has stood the test of time.

Finding Joy in Quick, Simple Meals

In today's fast-paced world, eating healthy often feels like an unattainable goal. That's where this cookbook becomes a game changer. Packed with recipes that take just 30 minutes or less to prepare, it shows you how to enjoy vibrant, flavorful meals without spending hours in the kitchen.

With minimal effort and maximum flavor, these recipes prove that cooking at home can be both quick and rewarding. From refreshing salads to hearty dinners, you'll learn how to transform simple ingredients into delicious dishes. Mediterranean cooking has never been more accessible—or enjoyable—even for the busiest of lifestyles.

The Benefits of Mediterranean Eating

The Mediterranean diet is renowned for its ability to nourish the body while pleasing the palate. This balanced approach to eating supports heart health, stabilizes energy levels, and reduces the risk of chronic diseases, including diabetes and obesity. Its combination of nutrient-dense foods and vibrant flavors ensures that every meal is as enjoyable as it is good for you.

By incorporating these recipes into your routine, you'll experience the incredible benefits of Mediterranean eating without complicated meal prep. These dishes will leave you feeling energized and satisfied, offering a sustainable and delicious way to maintain your health. With every bite, you'll be feeding your body and embracing a lifestyle of well-being.

Cooking for Wellness

Every ingredient in Mediterranean cooking plays a key role in promoting health and vitality. Olive oil, the backbone of this diet, is packed with heart-healthy monounsaturated fats and antioxidants. Fresh vegetables and fruits deliver essential vitamins, while lean proteins like fish and legumes provide lasting energy without weighing you down.

This cookbook is designed to help you make every meal a step toward better wellness. These recipes highlight the power of wholesome ingredients, showing that food can heal, nourish, and bring joy. Cooking Mediterranean-style is about more than feeding yourself—it's about investing in your overall health with every delicious dish.

Meals That Fit Your Schedule

One of the biggest barriers to healthy eating is time, but this cookbook eliminates that hurdle. Every recipe is crafted to fit seamlessly into your busy life, ensuring that you can enjoy wholesome, homemade meals in just 30 minutes. Whether it's a quick breakfast before work or a satisfying dinner after a long day, these dishes are designed with your schedule in mind.

With easy preparation and minimal cleanup, these recipes allow you to focus on what truly matters—enjoying your food and your time. Healthy eating becomes stress-free and enjoyable, proving that even the busiest days can include a moment of delicious self-care.

Fresh Ingredients, Bold Flavors

The magic of Mediterranean cooking lies in its simplicity. By using fresh, seasonal ingredients, every dish bursts with natural flavor and vibrant color. A squeeze of lemon, a drizzle of olive oil, or a handful of fresh herbs can elevate even the simplest ingredients into something extraordinary.

This book celebrates the bold flavors of Mediterranean cuisine while keeping the cooking process simple and enjoyable. Each recipe is a testament to the beauty of cooking with fresh produce, whole grains, and quality proteins. You'll discover how easy it is to make every meal both nutritious and unforgettable.

A Balance of Taste and Nutrition

The Mediterranean diet proves that healthy eating doesn't have to be bland or restrictive. These recipes strike the perfect balance between taste and nutrition, offering meals that satisfy your cravings while nourishing your body. From savory stews to refreshing salads, every dish is packed with flavor and essential nutrients.

This way of eating allows you to indulge in the richness of olive oil, the sweetness of ripe tomatoes, and the tang of fresh lemons while staying aligned with your health goals. It's a lifestyle that feels indulgent yet sustainable, making healthy eating something you'll look forward to every day.

Accessible for Beginners

Cooking Mediterranean-style is straightforward, making it perfect for both beginners and experienced chefs. This cookbook is filled with clear, step-by-step instructions that guide you through every recipe with ease. You don't need special skills or fancy equipment to create these delicious meals.

The ingredients are simple and easy to find, so there's no need to search for exotic items. With this book, you'll quickly gain confidence in the kitchen, learning how to prepare wholesome, flavorful dishes that your family will love. Mediterranean cooking is about enjoying the process as much as the final result.

Designed for Everyday Life

This cookbook is created for real life, offering recipes that fit seamlessly into your daily routine. With a 30-minute time frame, you can enjoy healthy, home-cooked meals without stress or hassle. The variety of dishes ensures that there's something for every mood and occasion.

From light salads to hearty mains, these recipes are versatile enough to suit busy weekdays or relaxed weekends. This book is your go-to resource for making healthy eating a regular, enjoyable part of your life. It's Mediterranean cooking made simple and practical.

Budget-Friendly and Sustainable

Eating well doesn't have to break the bank. This cookbook focuses on affordable ingredients that are easy to find and use. By prioritizing fresh produce, pantry staples, and simple proteins, it makes Mediterranean cooking accessible to everyone.

These recipes are also sustainable, encouraging the use of seasonal ingredients and minimizing food waste. By adopting this approach, you'll not only save money but also contribute to a healthier planet. Mediterranean cooking is about making the most of what you have while enjoying incredible meals.

Meals for Sharing

The heart of Mediterranean cooking lies in its ability to bring people together. Whether you're preparing a cozy dinner for your family or hosting friends for a celebration, these recipes are perfect for sharing. The warmth and flavors of these dishes invite connection and joy around the table.

Food has always been a way to strengthen bonds, and this cookbook embraces that tradition.

From hearty stews to vibrant salads, every recipe is designed to create moments of togetherness and happiness. Share these meals with your loved ones and enjoy the magic of Mediterranean cooking.

A Rich Culinary Tradition

Mediterranean cuisine is a tapestry of flavors and traditions, reflecting the diverse cultures of the region. From the tangy tzatziki of Greece to the aromatic spices of Morocco, this cookbook brings the rich heritage of Mediterranean cooking into your kitchen.

These recipes are your passport to a world of bold and vibrant flavors. They allow you to experience the unique culinary traditions of the Mediterranean while adapting them to your modern lifestyle. It's a celebration of history, culture, and incredible taste.

Flexible and Adaptable

Every recipe in this cookbook is a starting point for your creativity. You can adjust ingredients to suit your preferences, swap proteins, or experiment with new flavors. Mediterranean cooking is all about flexibility and making dishes your own.This approach ensures that cooking is never boring and always rewarding. Whether you're improvising with what's in your pantry or adding your personal twist to a classic recipe, these dishes are designed to inspire and delight.

Your Mediterranean Journey Begins Here

This cookbook is more than just a collection of recipes—it's your invitation to embrace a healthier, more fulfilling lifestyle inspired by the Mediterranean. In just 30 minutes a day, you'll create meals that nourish your body, satisfy your taste buds, and bring joy to your table, proving that healthy eating can be simple and enjoyable.

The Mediterranean diet isn't just about food; it's about savoring each moment, sharing meals with loved ones, and finding happiness in cooking. With vibrant flavors and fresh, wholesome ingredients, you'll discover how easy it is to make every meal feel special. Each recipe is designed to inspire confidence in the kitchen, even if you're just starting your cooking journey. As you explore the pages of this book, you'll uncover a lifestyle that prioritizes both health and flavor.

Let this book guide you through vibrant, wholesome recipes that fit effortlessly into your daily routine. Welcome to a journey of flavor, wellness, and connection—ready in just 30 minutes!

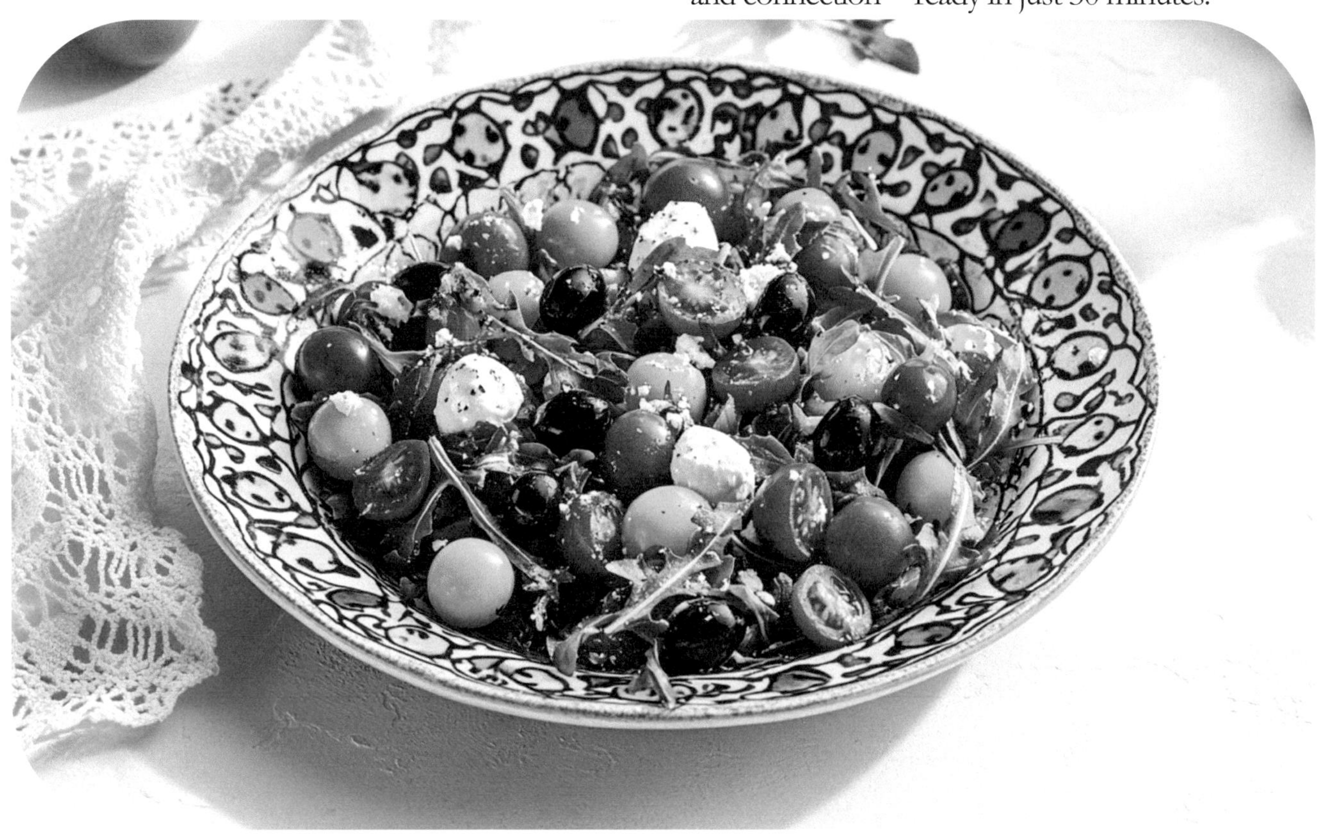

Chapter 1

BREAKFAST and APPETIZERS

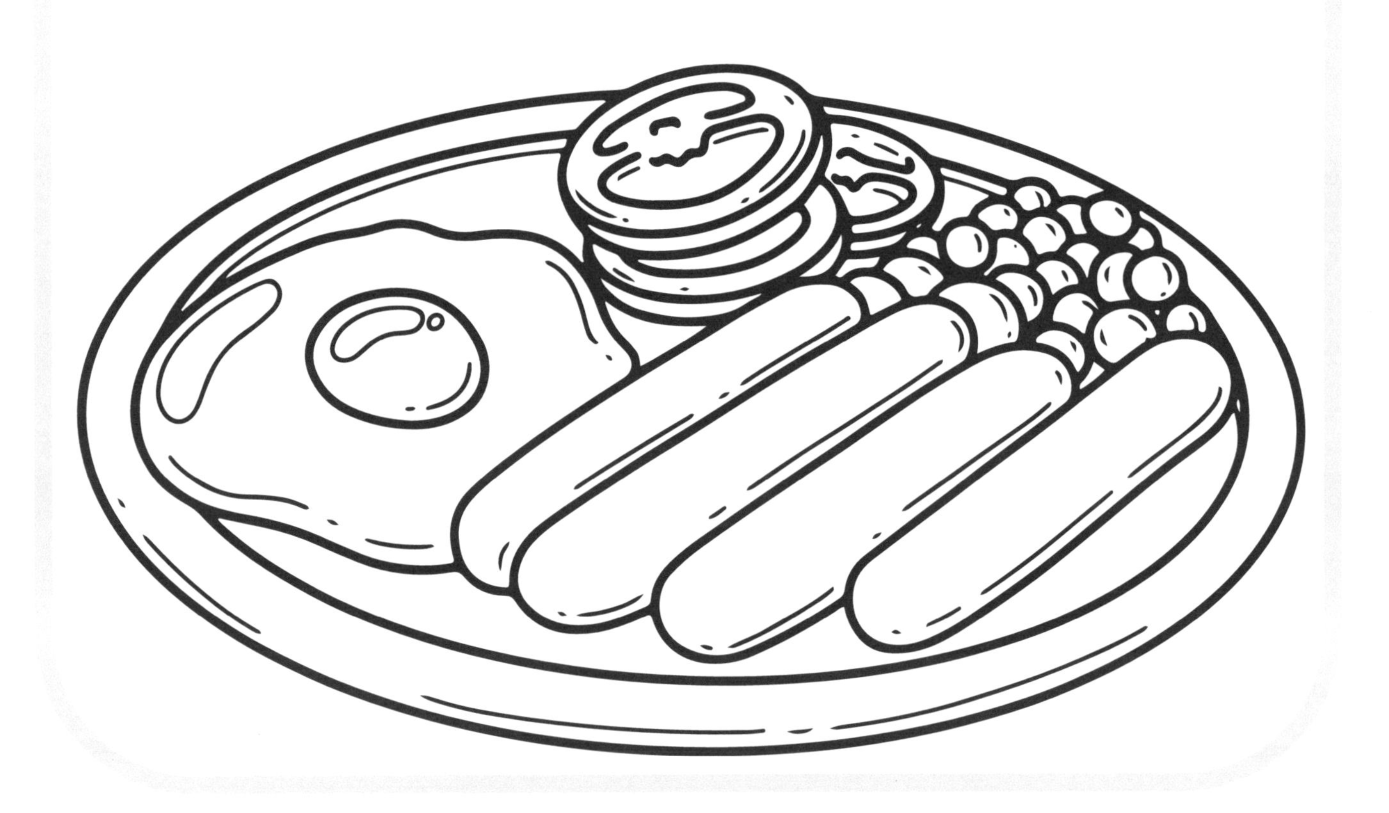

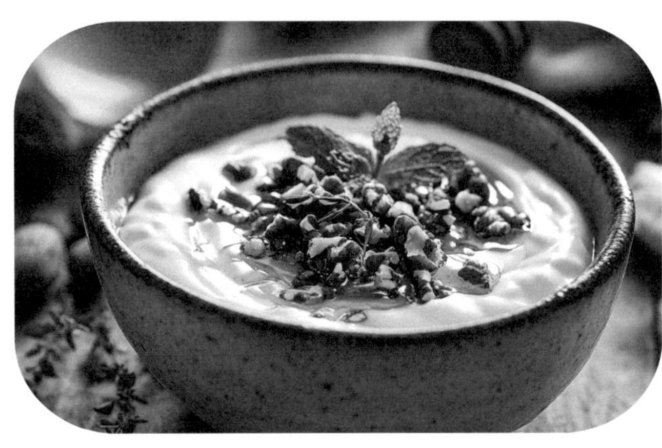

Greek Yogurt with Honey and Walnuts

PREPARATION TIME: 5 MINUTES

COOKING TIME: NONE

SERVES: 4

Nutrition Information (Per Serving):
220 Calories / 9g Fat / 25g Carbohydrates / 12g Protein / 65 mg Sodium / 20g Sugar

INGREDIENTS:

- 2 cups Greek yogurt
- 4 tablespoons honey
- 1/2 cup walnuts, chopped
- Optional: a pinch of ground cinnamon or a handful of fresh berries for garnish

DIRECTIONS:

1. Divide the Greek yogurt evenly into 4 serving bowls.
2. Drizzle 1 tablespoon of honey over each bowl of yogurt.
3. Sprinkle the chopped walnuts on top of each serving.
4. Optionally, add a pinch of cinnamon or fresh berries for extra flavor.
5. Serve immediately and enjoy!

TIP: Toast the walnuts briefly in a skillet over medium heat to enhance their flavor and add a crunchier texture.

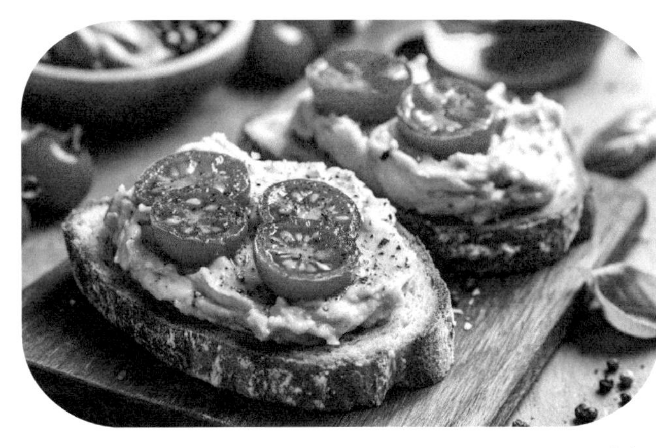

Avocado Toast with Olive Oil and Tomatoes

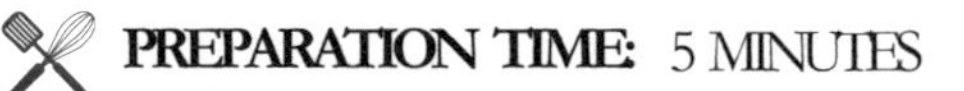

PREPARATION TIME: 5 MINUTES

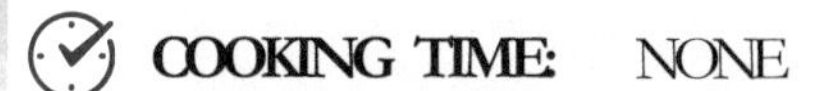

COOKING TIME: NONE

SERVES: 4

Nutrition Information (Per Serving):
190 Calories / 12g Fat / 16g Carbohydrates / 4g Protein / 180mg Sodium / 2g Sugar

INGREDIENTS:

- 2 ripe avocados
- 2 slices of whole-grain bread, or bread of your choice
- 1 cup cherry tomatoes, halved
- 4 tablespoons olive oil
- Salt and pepper to taste
- Optional: fresh basil leaves or a pinch of red pepper flakes for garnish

DIRECTIONS:

1. Toast the bread slices until golden and crisp.
2. Spread an even layer of mashed avocado over each slice of toast.
3. Top with halved cherry tomatoes, evenly distributed.
4. Drizzle 1 teaspoon of olive oil over each toast.
5. Sprinkle with sea salt and black pepper to taste.
6. Garnish with fresh basil leaves or a pinch of red pepper flakes if desired.
7. Serve immediately and enjoy this fresh, flavorful breakfast or snack!

TIP: For a richer flavor, try drizzling balsamic glaze or adding a sprinkle of crumbled feta cheese on top.

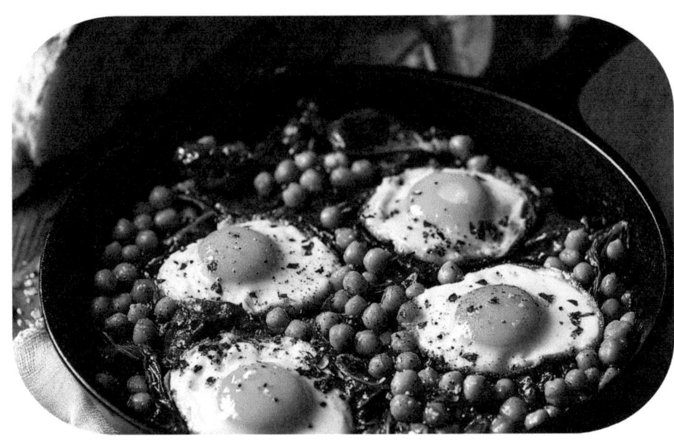

Mediterranean Breakfast Skillet

 **PREPARATION TIME:** 10 MINUTES

 **COOKING TIME:** 20 MINUTES

 **SERVES:** 4

Nutrition Information (Per Serving):
280 Calories / 12g Fat / 25g Carbohydrates / 14g Protein / 400mg Sodium / 3g Sugar

INGREDIENTS:

- 1 tablespoon olive oil
- 1 small red onion, finely chopped
- 2 garlic cloves, minced
- 1 teaspoon ground cumin
- 1/2 teaspoon smoked paprika
- 1 can (15 oz) chickpeas, drained and rinsed
- 4 cups fresh spinach leaves
- 4 large eggs
- Salt and pepper to taste
- 2 tablespoons fresh parsley, chopped

DIRECTIONS:

1. Heat olive oil in a large skillet over medium heat. Add the red onion and garlic, and sauté for 2-3 minutes until softened and fragrant.
2. Stir in the cumin and smoked paprika, cooking for 1 minute to release the spices' aroma.
3. Add the chickpeas and cook for 2-3 minutes, stirring to coat them with the spices.
4. Toss in the spinach and cook for 1-2 minutes, until just wilted.
5. Create four small wells in the skillet and crack an egg into each well. Cover the skillet and cook for 5-7 minutes, or until the egg whites are set but the yolks remain runny.
6. Season with salt and pepper to taste.
7. Sprinkle with chopped parsley before serving and enjoy warm.

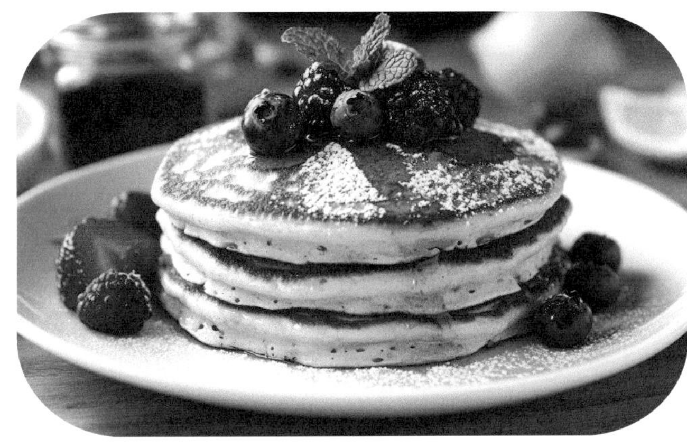

Lemon Ricotta Pancakes

 **PREPARATION TIME:** 10 MINUTES

 **COOKING TIME:** 15 MINUTES

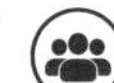 **SERVES:** 4

Nutrition Information (Per Serving):
250 Calories / 14g Fat / 22g Carbohydrates / 9g Protein / 270mg Sodium / 4g Sugar

INGREDIENTS:

- 2 cups ricotta cheese
- 4 large eggs
- 1 cup whole milk
- 2 tablespoons lemon zest (from 2 lemons)
- 4 tablespoons fresh lemon juice
- 2 cups all-purpose flour
- 2 tablespoons sugar
- 2 teaspoons baking powder
- 1/2 teaspoon salt
- Olive oil or butter for cooking
- Fresh berries and honey, for serving (optional)

DIRECTIONS:

1. In a large bowl, whisk together the ricotta cheese, eggs, milk, lemon zest, and lemon juice until smooth.
2. In a separate bowl, mix the flour, sugar, baking powder, and salt.
3. Gradually add the dry ingredients to the ricotta mixture, stirring until just combined; the batter will be thick.
4. Heat a non-stick skillet over medium heat and add a small amount of olive oil or butter.
5. Pour about 1/4 cup of batter onto the skillet for each pancake. Cook until bubbles form on the surface, about 2-3 minutes. Flip and cook for another 2-3 minutes or until golden brown.
6. Serve warm, topped with fresh berries and a drizzle of honey.

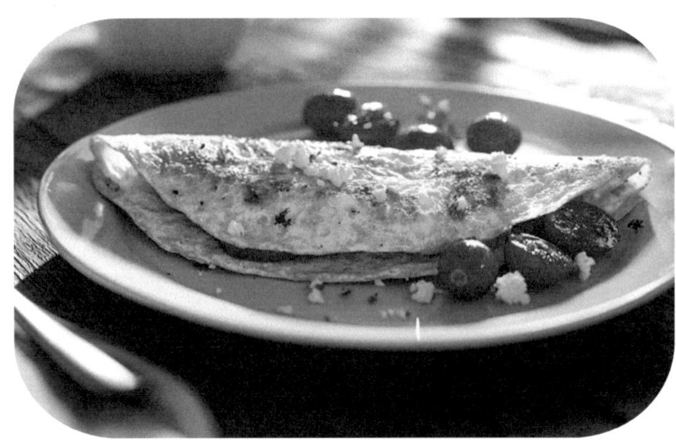

Tomato and Feta Omelette

PREPARATION TIME: 10 MINUTES

COOKING TIME: 10 MINUTES

SERVES: 4

Nutrition Information (Per Serving):
200 Calories / 14g Fat / 6g Carbohydrates / 12g Protein / 300mg Sodium / 3g Sugar

INGREDIENTS:

- 6-8 large eggs
- 1/2 cup crumbled feta cheese
- 1 cup cherry tomatoes, halved
- 2 tablespoons olive oil
- 1/4 cup chopped fresh basil (optional)
- Salt and pepper to taste

DIRECTIONS:

1. In a bowl, whisk the eggs until well combined. Season with salt and pepper.
2. Heat 1 tablespoon of olive oil in a non-stick pan over medium heat.
3. Pour in half of the egg mixture and cook for 2-3 minutes until the edges start to set.
4. Sprinkle half of the feta cheese and half of the cherry tomatoes over the eggs.
5. Cook for another 2-3 minutes until the eggs are fully set.
6. Fold the omelette in half and slide it onto a plate.
7. Repeat the process with the remaining egg mixture, feta, and tomatoes.
8. Garnish with fresh basil if desired, and serve immediately.

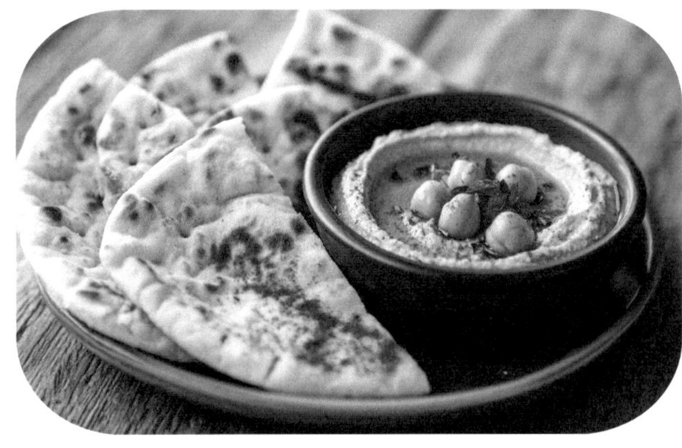

Simple Pita Bread with Hummus

PREPARATION TIME: 5 MINUTES

COOKING TIME: 5 MINUTES

SERVES: 4

Nutrition Information (Per Serving):
240 Calories / 9g Fat / 30g Carbohydrates / 7g Protein / 360mg Sodium / 1g Sugar

INGREDIENTS:

- 4 whole pita breads
- 1 cup hummus (see recipe on p.19)
- 2 tablespoons olive oil
- Paprika for garnish
- Fresh parsley leaves (optional)

DIRECTIONS:

1. Cut each pita bread in half and place the halves in a toaster. Toast on a low setting for 1-2 minutes or until the bread is warm and slightly crisp
2. Spoon the hummus into a serving bowl.
3. Drizzle olive oil over the hummus.
4. Sprinkle paprika over the top.
5. Garnish with parsley leaves.
6. Dip pita in hummus and enjoy!

TIP: Serve the hummus with a side of sliced cucumber and cherry tomatoes for a refreshing, crunchy accompaniment

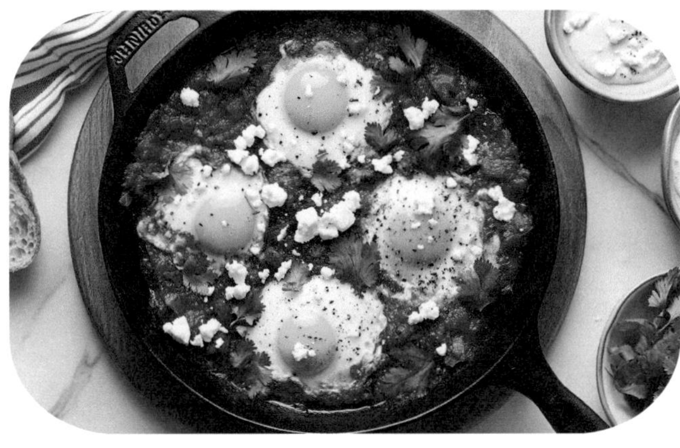

Simple Shakshuka

 **PREPARATION TIME:** 10 MINUTES

 **COOKING TIME:** 20 MINUTES

SERVES: 4

Nutrition Information (Per Serving):
250 Calories / 14g Fat / 20g Carbohydrates / 10g Protein / 450mg Sodium / 6g Sugar

INGREDIENTS:

- 4 large eggs
- 1 can (14 oz) diced tomatoes
- 1 red bell pepper, diced
- 1 onion, chopped
- 2 garlic cloves, minced
- 2 tablespoons olive oil
- 1 teaspoon ground cumin
- 1 teaspoon paprika
- Salt and pepper to taste
- Fresh cilantro for garnish

DIRECTIONS:

1. Heat olive oil in a large skillet over medium heat. Add the chopped onion and diced bell pepper, and cook until softened, about 5 minutes.
2. Stir in the minced garlic, ground cumin, and paprika, and cook for another minute until fragrant.
3. Pour in the diced tomatoes and bring the mixture to a simmer. Season with salt and pepper to taste.
4. Make four small wells in the tomato mixture, and crack an egg into each well.
5. Cover the skillet and cook for 7-10 minutes, or until the eggs are set to your liking.
6. Garnish with fresh cilantro and serve immediately with crusty bread.

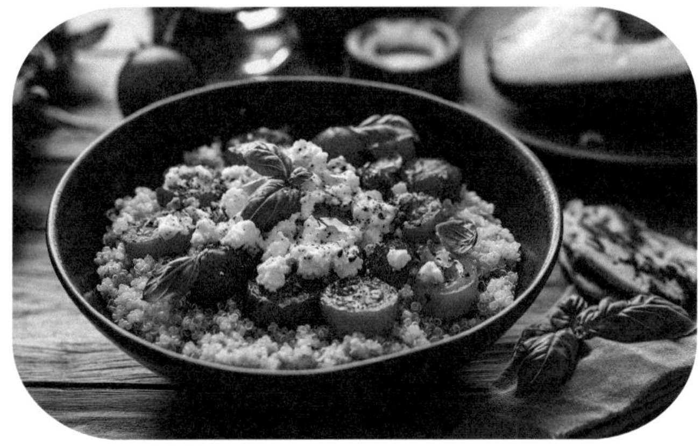

Quinoa Breakfast Bowl with Tomatoes

 **PREPARATION TIME:** 10 MINUTES

 **COOKING TIME:** 20 MINUTES

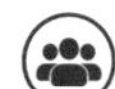 **SERVES:** 4

Nutrition Information (Per Serving):
230 Calories / 8g Fat / 30g Carbohydrates / 10g Protein / 300mg Sodium / 4g Sugar

INGREDIENTS:

- 1 cup quinoa
- 2 cups water
- 1 cup cherry tomatoes, halved
- 1/2 cup crumbled feta cheese
- 2 tablespoons olive oil
- Fresh basil for garnish
- Salt and pepper to taste

DIRECTIONS:

1. Rinse the quinoa under cold water. In a medium saucepan, bring the quinoa and water to a boil. Reduce heat, cover, and simmer for about 15 minutes, or until the water is absorbed and the quinoa is fluffy.
2. Divide the cooked quinoa into four bowls. Top each bowl with halved cherry tomatoes and crumbled feta cheese.
3. Drizzle with olive oil and season with salt and pepper.
4. Garnish with fresh basil leaves and serve warm.

TIP: Add a poached egg on top for extra protein and richness

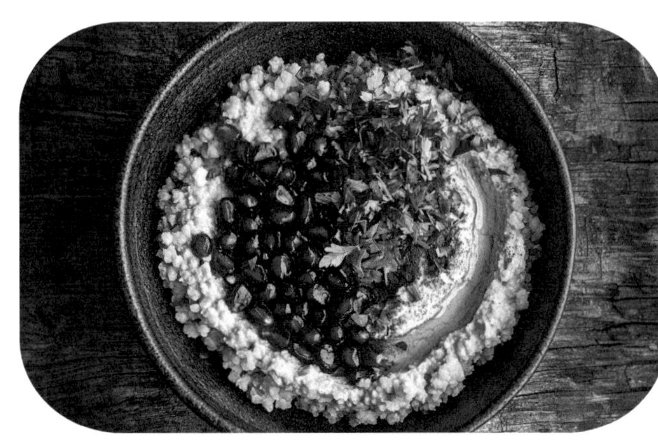

Hummus and Pomegranate Bulgur Bowl

PREPARATION TIME: 10 MINUTES

COOKING TIME: 15 MINUTES

SERVES: 4

Nutrition Information (Per Serving):
250 Calories / 8g Fat / 30g Carbohydrates / 12g Protein / 320mg Sodium / 2g Sugar

INGREDIENTS:

- 1 cup bulgur wheat
- 2 cups water or vegetable broth
- ½ cup hummus (see recipe on p.19)
- ½ cup pomegranate seeds
- 2 tablespoons fresh parsley, chopped
- 1 tablespoon olive oil
- 1 tablespoon lemon juice
- Salt and pepper to taste

DIRECTIONS:

1. In a small pot, bring the water or vegetable broth to a boil. Stir in the bulgur, cover, and reduce the heat to low. Simmer for 12-15 minutes, or until the bulgur is tender and the liquid is absorbed. Fluff with a fork and set aside.
2. Divide the cooked bulgur between two bowls. Drizzle with olive oil and lemon juice, and season with salt and pepper to taste.
3. Top each bowl with 2 tablespoons of hummus, sprinkle pomegranate seeds, and garnish with chopped parsley.
4. Serve warm or at room temperature.

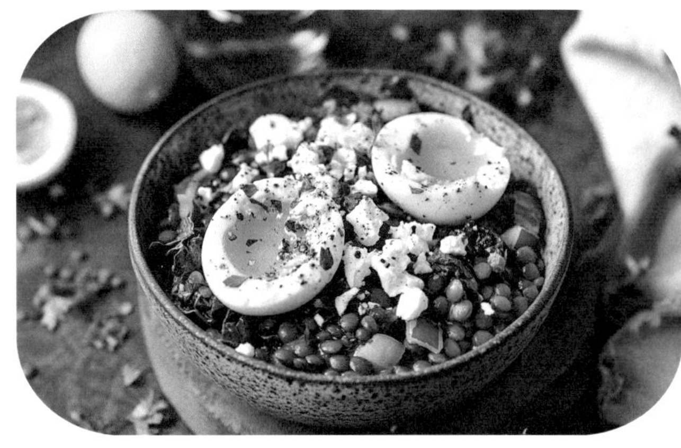

Warm Lentil Breakfast Bowl with Spinach

PREPARATION TIME: 10 MINUTES

COOKING TIME: 15 MINUTES

SERVES: 4

Nutrition Information (Per Serving):
250 Calories / 14g Fat / 22g Carbohydrates / 9g Protein / 270mg Sodium / 4g Sugar

INGREDIENTS:

- 1 cup dried lentils, rinsed
- 3 cups water or vegetable broth
- 2 cups fresh spinach leaves, chopped
- 1 small red onion, finely chopped
- 2 tablespoons olive oil
- 1 teaspoon ground cumin
- 1/2 teaspoon smoked paprika
- Juice of 1 lemon
- 1/4 cup crumbled feta cheese
- 2 tablespoons fresh parsley, chopped
- Salt and pepper to taste
- Optional: 4 soft-boiled eggs, halved

DIRECTIONS:

1. Cook lentils in water or broth for 12-15 minutes until tender, then drain.
2. Heat olive oil in a skillet over medium heat, sauté onions for 2-3 minutes, then stir in cumin and smoked paprika for 1 minute.
3. Add spinach and cook until wilted, about 1-2 minutes.
4. Mix in cooked lentils, squeeze lemon juice, and season with salt and pepper.
5. Divide into 4 bowls, top with crumbled feta, parsley, and optional soft-boiled eggs.
6. Serve warm and enjoy!

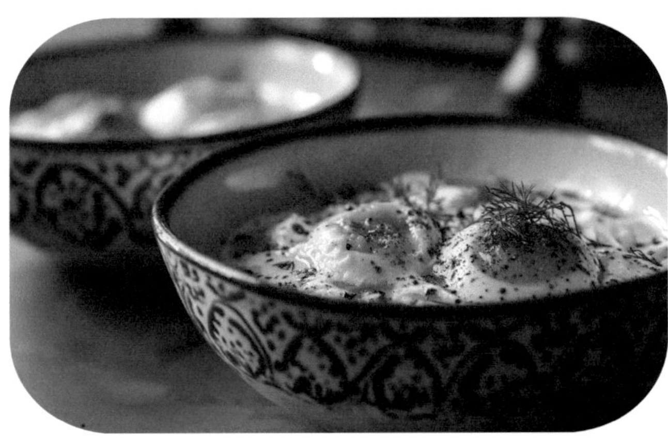

Çılbır (Turkish Poached Eggs with Yogurt)

PREPARATION TIME: 10 MINUTES

COOKING TIME: 10 MINUTES

SERVES: 4

Nutrition Information (Per Serving):
250 Calories / 18g Fat / 6g Carbohydrates / 14g Protein / 150mg Sodium / 3g Sugar

INGREDIENTS:

- 4 large eggs
- 2 cups Greek yogurt
- 2 garlic cloves, minced
- 2 tablespoons butter
- 1 teaspoon paprika (or Aleppo pepper)
- 1 tablespoon olive oil
- 1 tablespoon white vinegar
- Fresh dill or parsley for garnish
- Salt and pepper to taste

DIRECTIONS:

1. Mix Greek yogurt with minced garlic and a pinch of salt. Divide the yogurt mixture among four plates.
2. Simmer water with vinegar in a medium saucepan. Crack each egg into a small bowl, then gently slide it into the simmering water. Poach the eggs for 3-4 minutes until the whites are set but the yolks remain runny. Remove the eggs with a slotted spoon and place one egg on each plate of yogurt.
3. In a small skillet, melt butter over medium heat. Once it begins to foam, add paprika and stir for about 30 seconds until fragrant. Remove from heat and stir in olive oil.
4. Drizzle the butter and paprika sauce over the poached eggs and yogurt. Garnish with fresh dill or parsley. Serve immediately with crusty bread.

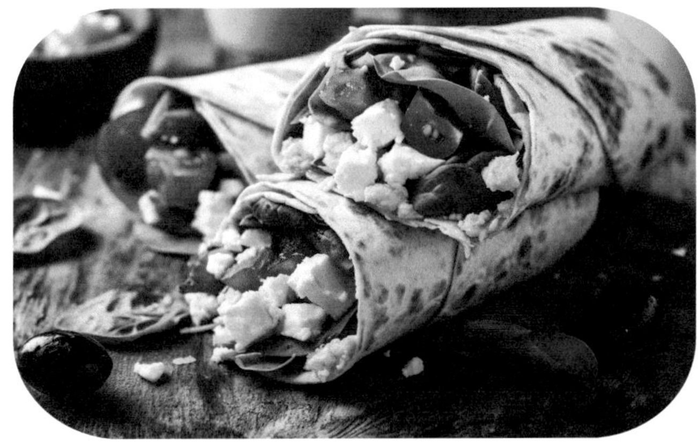

Mediterranean Breakfast Wrap

PREPARATION TIME: 10 MINUTES

COOKING TIME: 15 MINUTES

SERVES: 4

Nutrition Information (Per Serving):
280 Calories / 15g Fat / 25g Carbohydrates / 12g Protein / 500mg Sodium / 3g Sugar

INGREDIENTS:

- 4 large whole-wheat tortillas, or tortillas of your choice
- 1 cup hummus (see recipe on p.19)
- 1 cup fresh spinach leaves
- 1/2 cup diced tomatoes
- 1/2 cup crumbled feta cheese
- 1/4 cup sliced black olives (optional)
- Salt and pepper to taste

DIRECTIONS:

1. Lay the tortillas flat on a clean surface.
2. Evenly spread about 1/4 cup of hummus on each tortilla.
3. Layer fresh spinach leaves, diced tomatoes, and black olives (if using) on top of the hummus.
4. Sprinkle crumbled feta cheese over the vegetables.
5. Lightly season with salt and pepper.
6. Fold the sides of the tortilla inward, then roll it up tightly from the bottom to form a wrap.
7. Serve immediately or wrap in foil for an easy, portable breakfast.

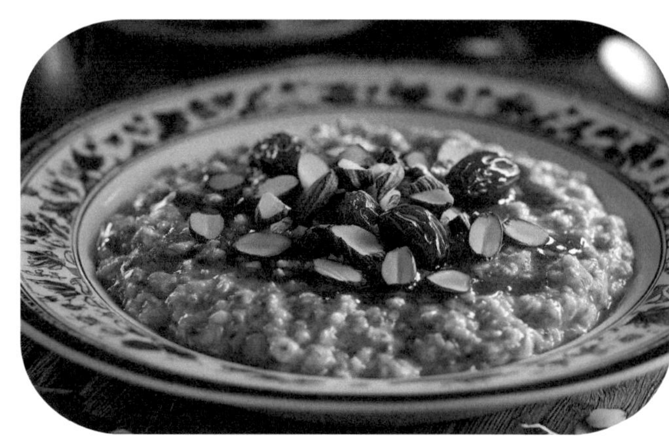

Mediterranean Oatmeal with Dates and Nuts

PREPARATION TIME: 5 MINUTES

COOKING TIME: 10 MINUTES

SERVES: 4

Nutrition Information (Per Serving):
350 Calories / 11g Fat / 60g Carbohydrates / 8g Protein / 90mg Sodium / 20g Sugar

INGREDIENTS:

- 2 cups rolled oats
- 4 cups water (or milk of your choice)
- 8 pitted dates, chopped
- 4 tablespoons chopped mixed nuts (such as almonds, walnuts, or pistachios)
- 2 tablespoons honey or maple syrup (optional, for extra sweetness)
- 1/2 teaspoon cinnamon (optional)
- A pinch of salt

DIRECTIONS:

1. In a medium saucepan, bring the water (or milk) to a boil.
2. Stir in the oats and reduce the heat to low. Simmer for 5-7 minutes, stirring occasionally, until the oats are tender and creamy.
3. Add the chopped dates, mixed nuts, cinnamon (if using), and a pinch of salt. Stir well to combine.
4. Cook for another 2-3 minutes to heat the dates and nuts through.
5. Remove from heat and drizzle honey or maple syrup on top if desired.
6. Divide the oatmeal into four bowls and serve warm.

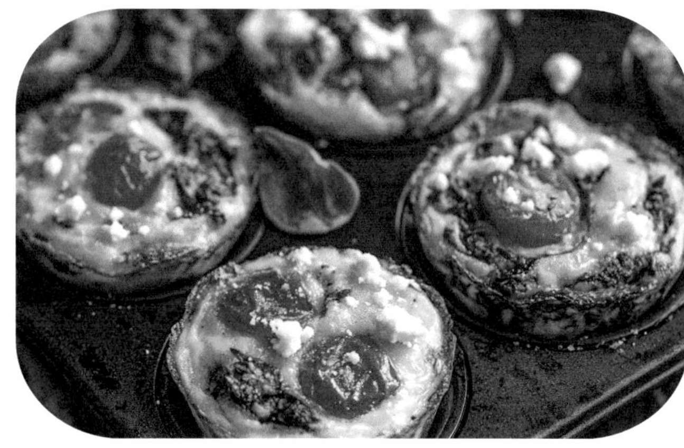

Spinach and Cheese Egg Muffins

PREPARATION TIME: 10 MINUTES

COOKING TIME: 20 MINUTES

SERVES: 4

Nutrition Information (Per Serving):
120 Calories / 8g Fat / 3g Carbohydrates / 9g Protein / 180mg Sodium / 1g Sugar

INGREDIENTS:

- 6 large eggs
- 1 cup fresh spinach, chopped
- 4 tablespoons feta cheese, crumbled
- 4 tablespoons cherry tomatoes, diced
- Salt and pepper, to taste

DIRECTIONS:

1. Preheat your oven to 350°F (175°C). Lightly grease a muffin tin or use silicone muffin cups.
2. In a medium bowl, whisk together the eggs with a pinch of salt and pepper. Stir in the chopped spinach, diced cherry tomatoes, and crumbled feta cheese.
3. Pour the egg mixture evenly into 6-8 muffin cups, filling them about three-quarters full.
4. Place the muffin tin in the preheated oven and bake for 15-20 minutes, or until the egg muffins are set and slightly golden on top.
5. Let the muffins cool slightly before removing them from the tin. Serve warm or at room temperature.

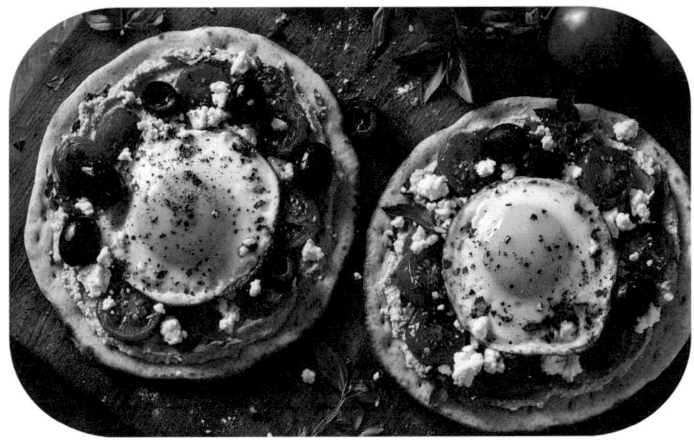

Mediterranean Breakfast Pizza

 **PREPARATION TIME:** 10 MINUTES

 **COOKING TIME:** 10 MINUTES

SERVES: 4

Nutrition Information (Per Serving):
320 Calories / 16g Fat / 30g Carbohydrates / 12g Protein / 400mg Sodium / 4g Sugar

INGREDIENTS:

- 4 whole-wheat pita breads
- 1/2 cup hummus (see recipe on p.19)
- 1/2 cup cherry tomatoes, halved
- 1/4 cup sliced black olives
- 1/4 cup crumbled feta cheese
- 4 large eggs
- 2 tablespoons olive oil
- Fresh basil or parsley for garnish
- Salt and pepper to taste

DIRECTIONS:

1. Preheat your oven to 375°F (190°C).
2. Place the pita breads on a baking sheet. Spread a layer of hummus evenly over each pita.
3. Top with cherry tomatoes, black olives, and crumbled feta cheese.
4. Drizzle a little olive oil over the toppings and season with salt and pepper.
5. Make a small well in the center of each pita and crack an egg into each well.
6. Bake in the preheated oven for 8-10 minutes, or until the egg whites are set and the yolks are cooked to your liking.
7. Garnish with fresh basil or parsley before serving.

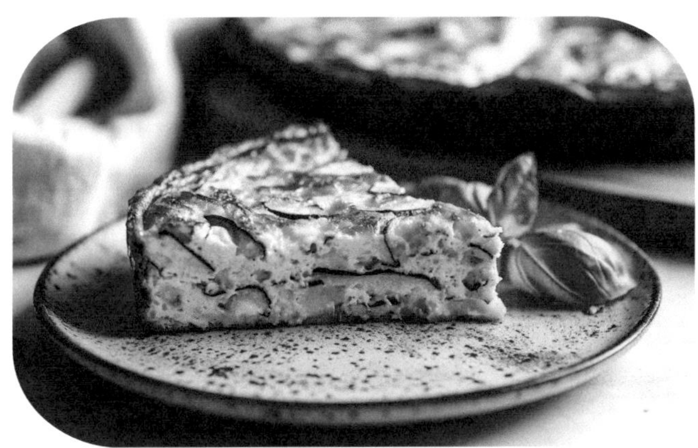

Baked Zucchini Frittata

 **PREPARATION TIME:** 5 MINUTES

 **COOKING TIME:** 25 MINUTES

 **SERVES:** 4

Nutrition Information (Per Serving):
180 Calories / 12g Fat / 7g Carbohydrates / 10g Protein / 250mg Sodium / 2g Sugar

INGREDIENTS:

- 4 large eggs
- 2 medium zucchinis, grated
- 1/2 cup grated Parmesan cheese
- 1/4 cup chopped fresh basil
- 2 tablespoons olive oil
- Salt and pepper to taste

DIRECTIONS:

1. Preheat your oven to 375°F (190°C).
2. In a large bowl, beat the eggs. Mix in the grated zucchini, Parmesan, basil, salt, and pepper.
3. Heat the olive oil in an ovenproof skillet over medium heat. Pour the egg mixture into the skillet and cook for 5 minutes until the edges start to set.
4. Transfer the skillet to the oven and bake for 20 minutes, or until the frittata is set and lightly golden.
5. Let cool slightly, slice into wedges, and serve warm or at room temperature.

TIP: Pair your frittata with a light drizzle of garlic aioli or a dollop of pesto for added flavor.

Chapter 2

SAUCES and DIPS

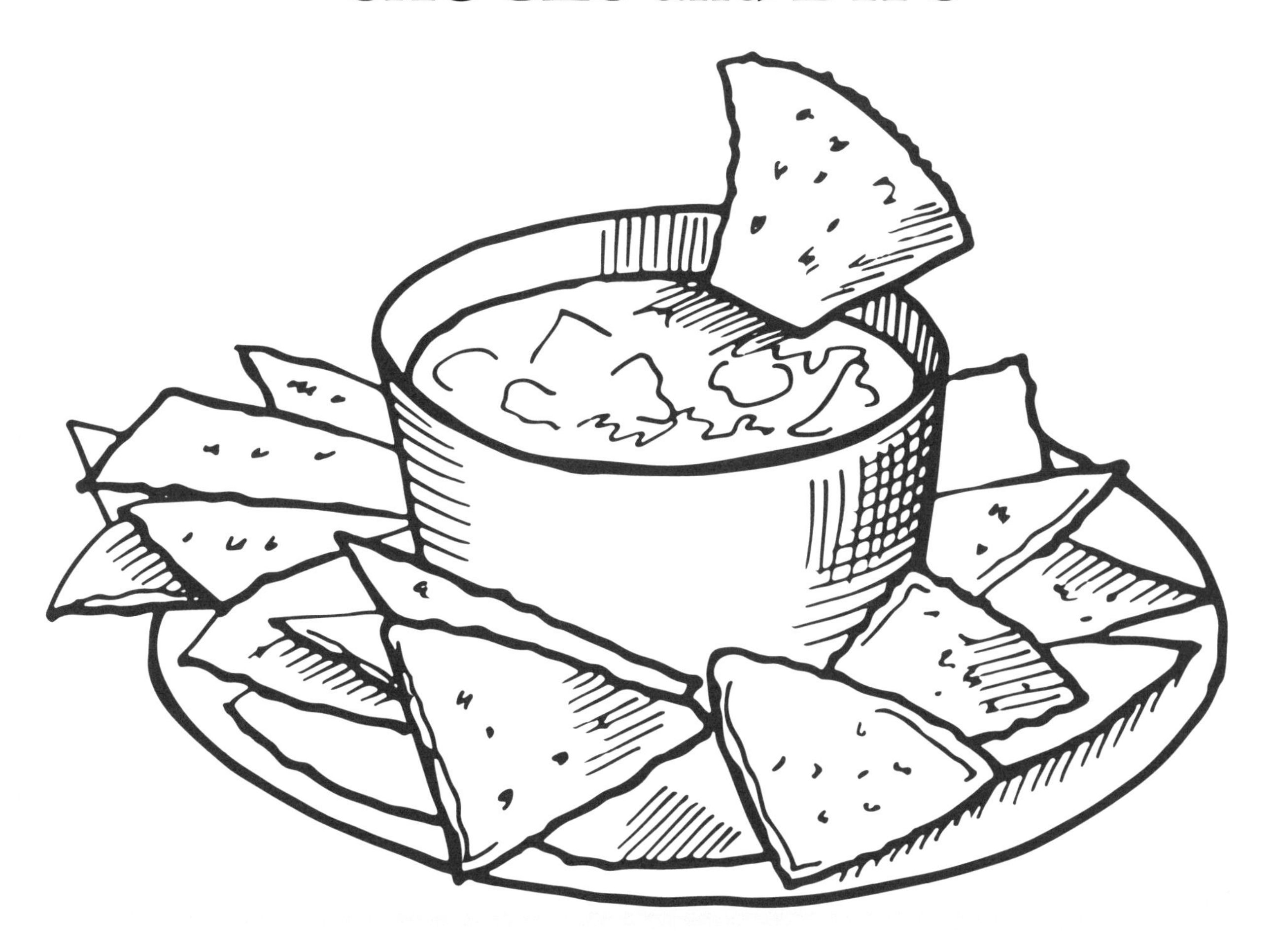

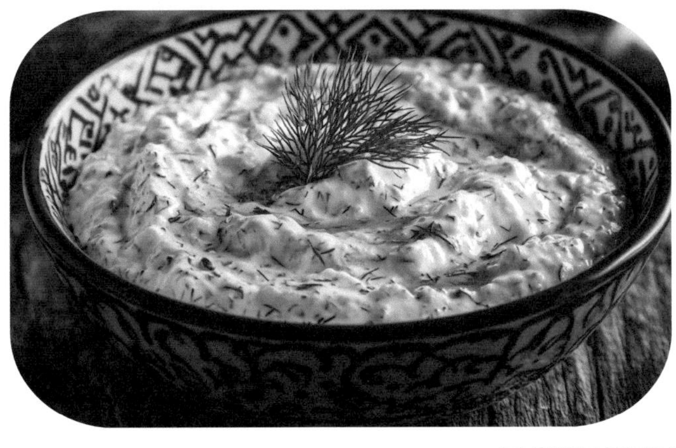

Greek Tzatziki Dip

PREPARATION TIME: 10 MINUTES

COOKING TIME: NONE

CHILLING TIME: 20 MINUTES

SERVES: 4

Nutrition Information (Per Serving):
100 Calories / 6g Fat / 6g Carbohydrates / 4g Protein / 60mg Sodium / 4g Sugar

INGREDIENTS:

- 1 cup Greek yogurt
- 1 cucumber, grated and drained
- 2 garlic cloves, minced
- 1 tablespoon olive oil
- 1 tablespoon fresh lemon juice
- 1 tablespoon chopped fresh dill
- Salt and pepper to taste

DIRECTIONS:

1. Grate the cucumber and squeeze out the excess water using a clean kitchen towel or paper towels.
2. In a medium bowl, combine the Greek yogurt, grated cucumber, minced garlic, olive oil, and lemon juice.
3. Stir in the chopped dill and season with salt and pepper.
4. Mix well until all ingredients are fully combined.
5. Refrigerate for at least 20 minutes to allow the flavors to meld.
6. Serve chilled with pita bread, fresh vegetables, or as a sauce for grilled meats.

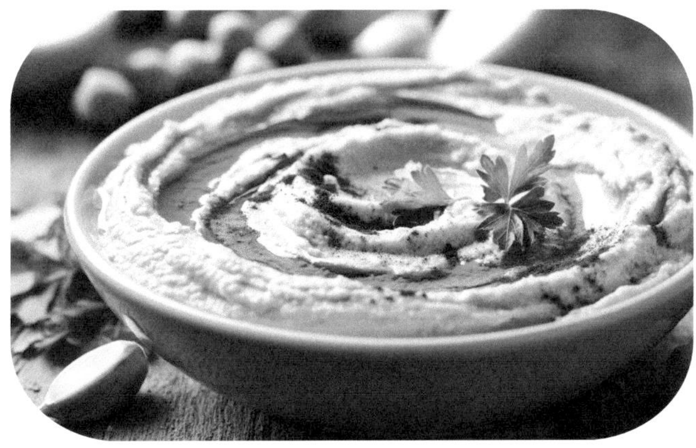

Hummus with Olive Oil and Paprika

PREPARATION TIME: 10 MINUTES

COOKING TIME: 5 MINUTES

SERVES: 4

Nutrition Information (Per Serving):
180 Calories / 12g Fat / 14g Carbohydrates / 6g Protein / 240mg Sodium / 1g Sugar

INGREDIENTS:

- 1 can (15 oz) chickpeas, drained and rinsed
- 1/4 cup tahini sauce (see recipe on p.20)
- 2 tablespoons lemon juice
- 1 garlic clove, minced
- 2 tablespoons extra virgin olive oil, plus more for drizzling
- 1/2 teaspoon ground cumin
- Salt to taste
- Water, as needed for consistency
- 1/2 teaspoon paprika, for garnish

DIRECTIONS:

1. In a food processor, combine the chickpeas, tahini, lemon juice, garlic, olive oil, cumin, and salt.
2. Blend until smooth, adding water a tablespoon at a time until desired consistency is reached.
3. Transfer the hummus to a serving bowl and drizzle with olive oil.
4. Sprinkle with paprika for garnish.
5. Serve with pita bread, vegetables, or as desired.

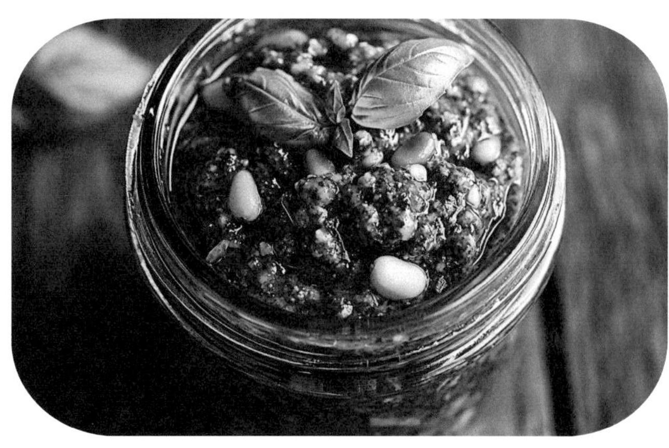

Simple Pesto

PREPARATION TIME: 10 MINUTES

COOKING TIME: NONE

SERVES: 4

Nutrition Information (Per Serving):
200 Calories / 20g Fat / 2g Carbohydrates / 3g Protein / 150mg Sodium / 0g Sugar

INGREDIENTS:

- 2 cups fresh basil leaves
- 1/2 cup extra virgin olive oil
- 1/3 cup pine nuts or walnuts
- 2 cloves garlic, minced
- 1/2 cup grated Parmesan cheese
- Salt and pepper to taste
- Optional: a squeeze of lemon juice

DIRECTIONS:

1. In a food processor, combine the basil leaves, nuts, and garlic. Pulse until finely chopped.
2. While the processor is running, slowly drizzle in the olive oil until the mixture is smooth.
3. Add the grated Parmesan cheese, and pulse until combined.
4. Season with salt, pepper, and optionally, a squeeze of lemon juice to brighten the flavor.
5. Serve immediately or store in an airtight container in the refrigerator.

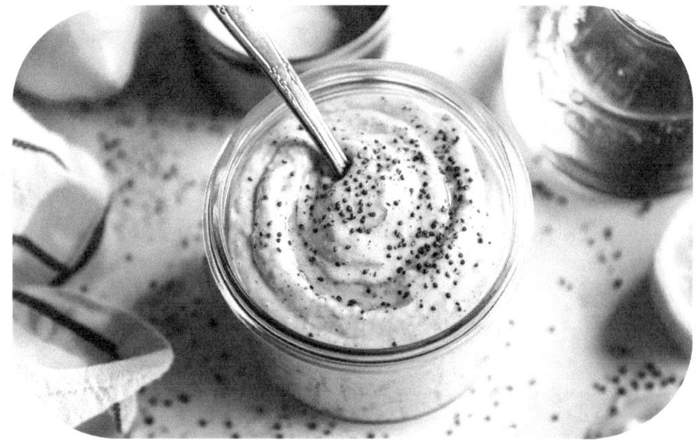

Tahini Sauce

PREPARATION TIME: 10 MINUTES

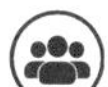

COOKING TIME: NONE

SERVES: 4

Nutrition Information (Per Serving):
160 Calories / 14g Fat / 5g Carbohydrates / 4g Protein / 100mg Sodium / 0g Sugar

INGREDIENTS:

- 1/2 cup crushed sesame seeds
- 1/4 cup water (adjust for desired consistency)
- 2 tablespoons lemon juice
- 1 garlic clove, minced
- Salt to taste
- Optional: a pinch of ground cumin or paprika

DIRECTIONS:

1. In a bowl, whisk together the crushed sesame seeds and lemon juice until well combined.
2. Gradually add water, whisking until the sauce reaches your desired consistency.
3. Stir in the minced garlic and salt to taste.
4. Optionally, add a pinch of cumin or paprika for extra flavor.
5. Serve immediately or refrigerate in an airtight container.

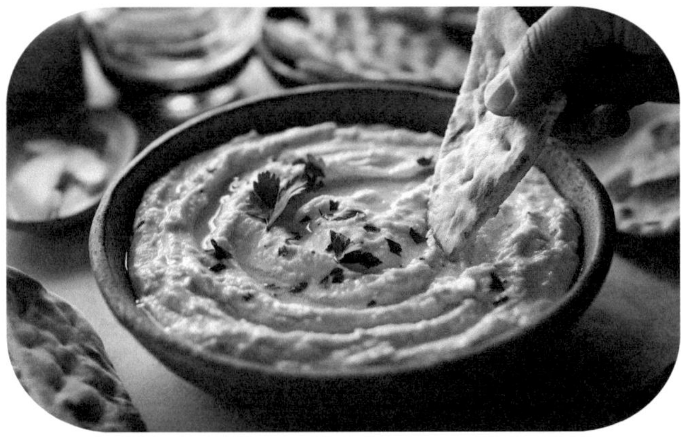

Skordalia (Garlic-Potato Dip)

PREPARATION TIME: 15 MINUTES

COOKING TIME: 10 MINUTES

SERVES: 4

Nutrition Information (Per Serving):
180 Calories / 12g Fat / 15g Carbohydrates / 3g Protein / 200mg Sodium / 2g Sugar

INGREDIENTS:

- 4 medium potatoes, peeled and chopped
- 4 cloves garlic, minced
- 1/4 cup extra virgin olive oil
- 2 tablespoons lemon juice
- 1/4 cup warm water
- Salt and pepper to taste
- Optional: 2 tablespoons white wine vinegar

DIRECTIONS:

1. Boil the chopped potatoes in salted water for about 10 minutes, or until tender. Drain and set aside.
2. In a food processor, combine the garlic, olive oil, lemon juice, and warm water.
3. Add the boiled potatoes to the processor and blend until smooth and creamy.
4. Season with salt and pepper to taste.
5. Optionally, add white wine vinegar for a tangier flavor.
6. Serve as a dip with bread, vegetables, or as a sauce for grilled meats.

TIP: For extra flavor, add a handful of chopped fresh herbs like parsley or dill to the dip.

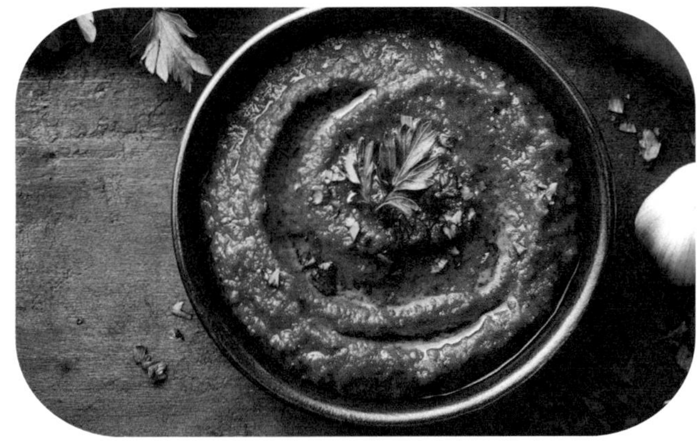

Roasted Red Pepper Dip

PREPARATION TIME: 5 MINUTES

COOKING TIME: NONE (+ time for roasting peppers if cooking them)

SERVES: 4

Nutrition Information (Per Serving):
150 Calories / 10g Fat / 13g Carbohydrates / 3g Protein / 200mg Sodium / 4g Sugar

INGREDIENTS:

- 2 large roasted red peppers (jarred or homemade)
- 1/4 cup tahini sauce (see recipe on p.20)
- 2 tablespoons lemon juice
- 1 garlic clove, minced
- 2 tablespoons extra virgin olive oil
- 1/2 teaspoon ground cumin
- Salt and pepper to taste
- 1/4 teaspoon smoked paprika (optional)
- Fresh parsley for garnish (optional)

DIRECTIONS:

1. If making homemade roasted peppers, preheat the oven to 425°F (220°C). Place a whole red pepper on a lined baking sheet and bake for 20-25 minutes, turning occasionally, until the skin is charred and blistered. Let it cool, then peel off the skin and remove the seeds.
2. In a food processor, combine the roasted red peppers, tahini, lemon juice, garlic, olive oil, cumin, salt, and pepper.
3. Blend until smooth, adjusting seasoning to taste.
4. Transfer the dip to a serving bowl and drizzle with olive oil.
5. Optionally, sprinkle with smoked paprika and garnish with fresh parsley.
6. Serve with pita bread, crackers, or fresh vegetables.

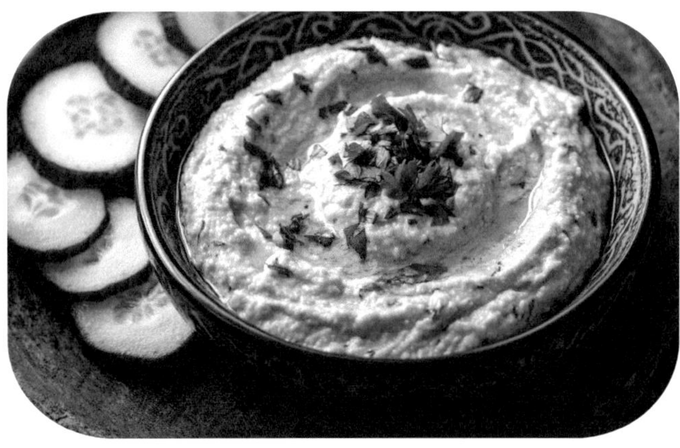

Baba Ganoush

PREPARATION TIME: 5 MINUTES

COOKING TIME: 20-25 MINUTES

SERVES: 4

Nutrition Information (Per Serving):
120 Calories / 10g Fat / 8g Carbohydrates / 2g Protein / 150mg Sodium / 3g Sugar

INGREDIENTS:

- 2 large eggplants
- 1/4 cup tahini sauce (see recipe on p.20)
- 2 tablespoons lemon juice
- 2 cloves garlic, minced
- 2 tablespoons extra virgin olive oil, plus more for drizzling
- Salt and pepper to taste
- Optional: 1/4 teaspoon ground cumin
- Fresh parsley for garnish

DIRECTIONS:

1. Preheat your oven to 400°F (200°C).
2. Pierce the eggplants with a fork and place them on a baking sheet. Roast in the oven for about 20-25 minutes, turning occasionally, until the skin is charred and the flesh is soft.
3. Once roasted, let the eggplants cool slightly, then peel off the skin and discard it. Place the flesh in a colander to drain any excess liquid.
4. In a food processor, combine the roasted eggplant flesh, tahini, lemon juice, garlic, olive oil, salt, and pepper. Add ground cumin if desired.
5. Blend until smooth and creamy, adjusting seasoning to taste.
6. Transfer the Baba Ganoush to a serving bowl, drizzle with a little olive oil, and garnish with fresh parsley.
7. Serve with pita bread, crackers, or fresh vegetables.

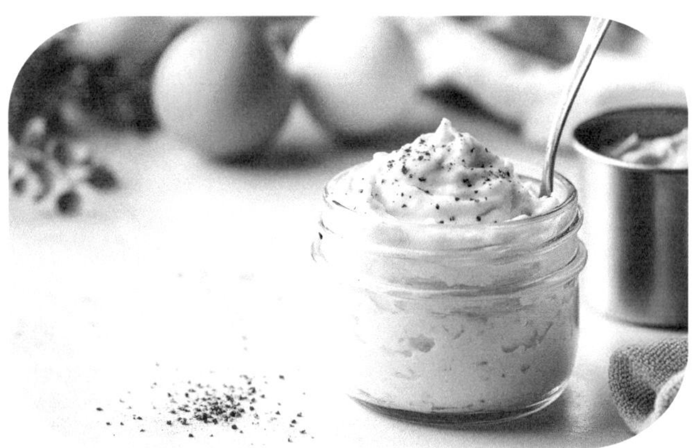

Aioli (Mediterranean Garlic Mayonnaise)

PREPARATION TIME: 10 MINUTES

COOKING TIME: NONE

SERVES: 4

Nutrition Information (Per Serving):
180 Calories / 18g Fat / 1g Carbohydrates / 1g Protein / 120mg Sodium / 0g Sugar

INGREDIENTS:

- 4 cloves garlic, minced
- 1 large egg yolk, at room temperature
- 1 cup extra virgin olive oil
- 1 tablespoon lemon juice
- 1 teaspoon Dijon mustard (optional, for stability)
- Salt to taste
- Optional: a pinch of ground black pepper or paprika

DIRECTIONS:

1. In a medium bowl, whisk together the minced garlic, egg yolk, and Dijon mustard (if using) until well combined.
2. Begin adding the olive oil very slowly, almost drop by drop, while continuously whisking. This allows the oil to emulsify with the egg yolk, creating a thick, creamy sauce.
3. As the mixture thickens, you can gradually increase the speed at which you add the olive oil, but continue whisking vigorously to maintain the emulsion.
4. Once all the oil is incorporated, stir in the lemon juice and season with salt. Add a pinch of ground black pepper or paprika if desired.
5. Taste and adjust the seasoning if necessary.
6. Transfer the aioli to a serving dish and serve immediately or refrigerate until ready to use.

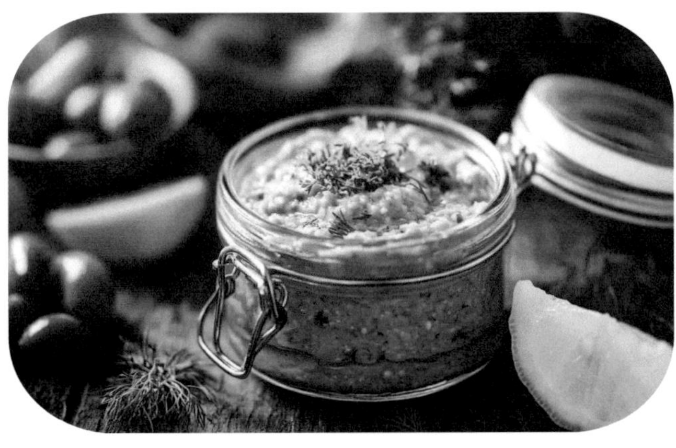

Taramosalata (Greek Caviar Spread)

PREPARATION TIME: 15 MINUTES

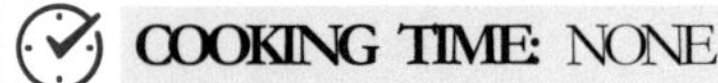

COOKING TIME: NONE

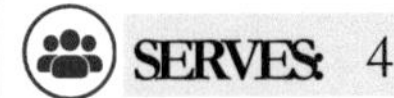

SERVES: 4

Nutrition Information (Per Serving):
190 Calories / 14g Fat / 12g Carbohydrates / 4g Protein / 300mg Sodium / 1g Sugar

INGREDIENTS:

- 1/2 cup tarama (fish roe, typically from carp or cod)
- 2 slices of stale white bread, crusts removed
- 1 small onion, grated or finely chopped
- 1/2 cup olive oil
- 2 tablespoons lemon juice
- 1-2 tablespoons water (optional, for adjusting consistency)
- Salt and pepper to taste

DIRECTIONS:

1. Soak the bread slices in water for a few minutes, then squeeze out the excess water.
2. In a food processor, combine the tarama (fish roe), soaked bread, grated onion, and lemon juice. Blend until smooth.
3. Slowly add the olive oil in a steady stream while the food processor is running, allowing the mixture to emulsify and become creamy.
4. If the mixture is too thick, you can add 1-2 tablespoons of water to adjust the consistency.
5. Season with salt and pepper to taste, blending again to incorporate.
6. Transfer the taramosalata to a serving bowl and garnish with a drizzle of olive oil and a sprinkle of fresh herbs, if desired.
7. Serve with pita bread, fresh vegetables, or as part of a mezze platter.

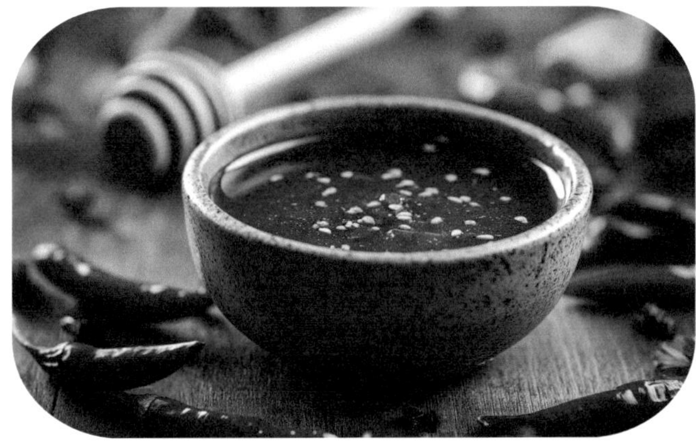

Homemade Hot Honey

PREPARATION TIME: 5 MINUTES

COOKING TIME: 10 MINUTES

SERVES: 1 Cup (approximately 16 tablespoons)

Nutrition Information (Per Tablespoon):
60 Calories / 0g Fat / 17g Carbohydrates / 0g Protein / 0mg Sodium / 17g Sugar

INGREDIENTS:

- 1 cup honey
- 1-2 tablespoons crushed red pepper flakes (adjust to taste)
- 1 teaspoon apple cider vinegar (optional, for a tangy kick)

DIRECTIONS:

1. In a small saucepan, combine the honey and crushed red pepper flakes.
2. Heat over low heat, stirring occasionally, for about 10 minutes. Do not let the honey boil; you want to gently warm it to extract the heat from the pepper flakes.
3. If you like a bit of tanginess, stir in the apple cider vinegar after removing the honey from the heat (add vinegar (Optional))
4. Allow the honey to cool slightly, then strain it through a fine-mesh sieve to remove the pepper flakes (optional, if you prefer a smoother texture).
5. Transfer the hot honey to a clean jar and store it at room temperature.

TIP: Drizzle over pizza, fried chicken, roasted vegetables, or use it in salad dressings.

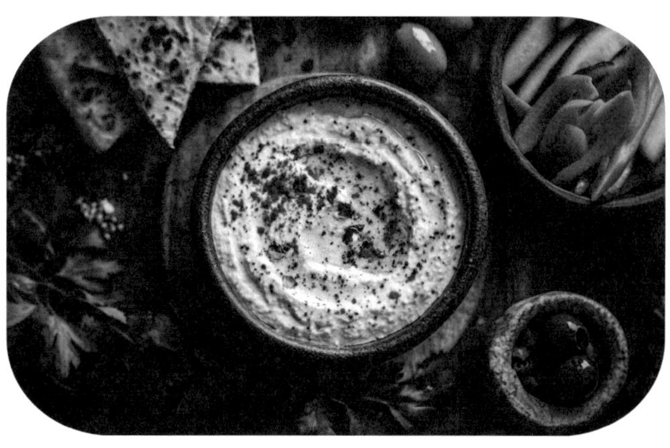

Tirokafteri (Spicy Feta Dip)

PREPARATION TIME: 5 MINUTES

COOKING TIME: NONE (+ time for roasting peppers if cooking them)

SERVES: 4

Nutrition Information (Per Serving):
150 Calories / 12g Fat / 4g Carbohydrates / 6g Protein / 480mg Sodium / 2g Sugar

INGREDIENTS:

- 1 cup feta cheese, crumbled
- 1/4 cup Greek yogurt
- 1-2 tablespoons olive oil
- 1 roasted red pepper, chopped (from a jar or freshly roasted)
- 1 small chili pepper (or 1/2 teaspoon red chili flakes, for less heat)
- Juice of 1/2 lemon
- 1 garlic clove, minced
- 1/4 teaspoon smoked paprika
- Salt to taste (optional, depending on the saltiness of the feta)

DIRECTIONS:

1. If making homemade roasted peppers, preheat the oven to 425°F (220°C). Place a whole red pepper on a lined baking sheet and bake for 20-25 minutes, turning occasionally, until the skin is charred and blistered. Let it cool, then peel off the skin and remove the seeds.
2. In a food processor or blender, combine feta cheese, Greek yogurt, olive oil, roasted red pepper, chili pepper, lemon juice, minced garlic, and smoked paprika.
3. Blend until smooth and creamy. Adjust the consistency by adding a little more olive oil or yogurt if needed.
4. Taste and add salt if necessary, depending on the saltiness of the feta.
5. Transfer to a serving bowl and drizzle with olive oil.
6. Serve immediately with pita bread, fresh vegetables, or crackers for dipping.

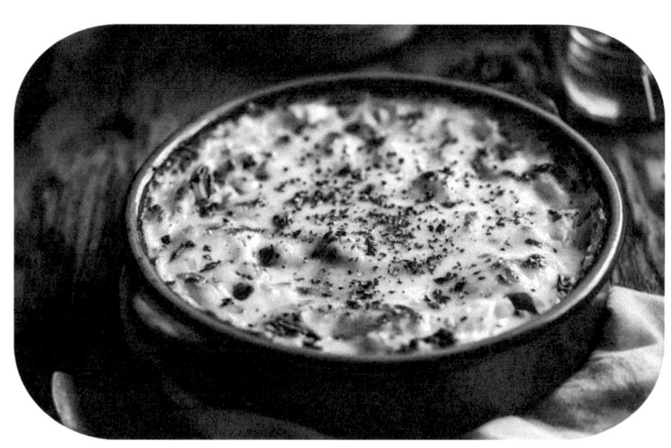

Artichoke and Spinach Dip

PREPARATION TIME: 10 MINUTES

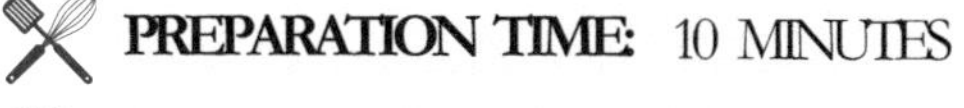

COOKING TIME: 15 MINUTES

SERVES: 4

Nutrition Information (Per Tablespoon):
120 Calories / 8g Fat / 10g Carbohydrates / 3g Protein / 220mg Sodium / 2g Sugar

INGREDIENTS:

- 1 cup canned or jarred artichoke hearts, drained and chopped
- 1 cup fresh spinach leaves, chopped
- 1/2 cup Greek yogurt
- 1/2 cup cream cheese, softened
- 1/4 cup grated Parmesan cheese
- 1/2 cup shredded mozzarella cheese
- 2 garlic cloves, minced
- 1 tablespoon olive oil
- Salt and pepper to taste

DIRECTIONS:

1. Preheat your oven to 375°F (190°C).
2. Heat olive oil in a skillet over medium heat. Add garlic and sauté for 1-2 minutes until fragrant. Stir in the chopped spinach and cook for 2-3 minutes until wilted.
3. In a mixing bowl, combine the artichoke hearts, sautéed spinach, Greek yogurt, cream cheese, Parmesan cheese, and half of the mozzarella cheese. Mix until well blended.
4. Transfer the mixture to a small baking dish and sprinkle the remaining mozzarella cheese on top.
5. Bake in the preheated oven for 12-15 minutes, or until the dip is bubbling and the cheese on top is golden.
6. Serve warm with pita chips, fresh vegetables, or crusty bread for dipping.

Chapter 3

SALADS and SOUPS

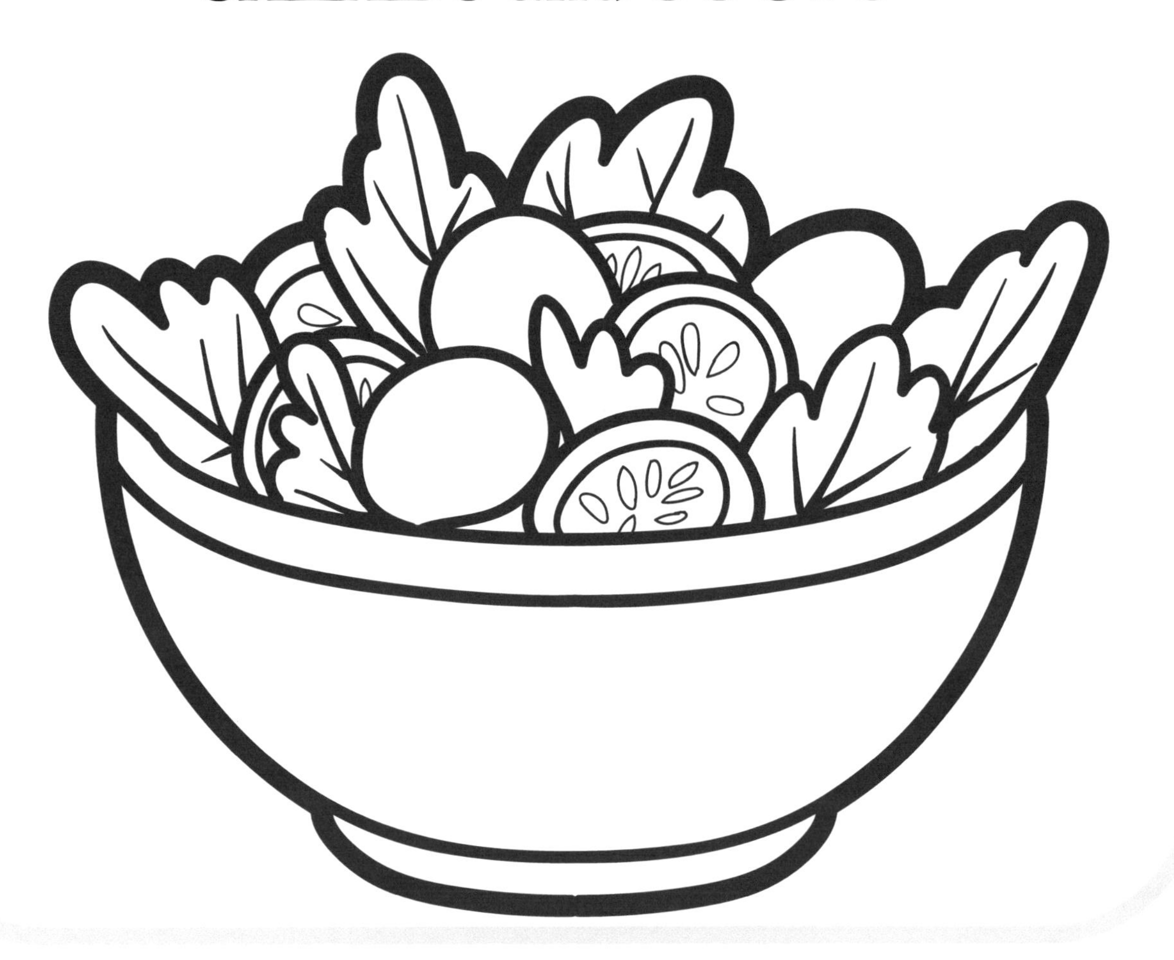

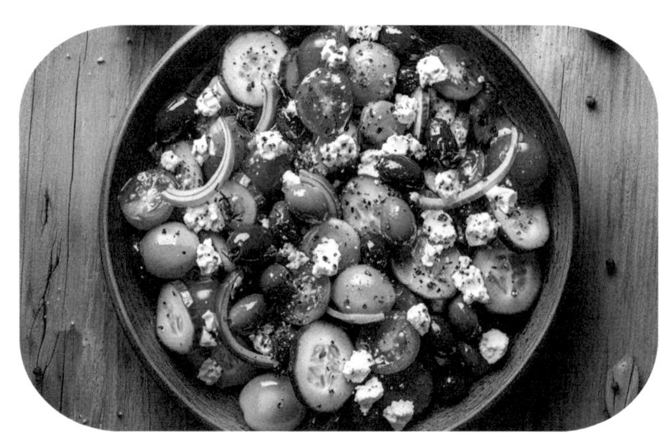

Greek Salad

PREPARATION TIME: 10 MINUTES

COOKING TIME: NONE

SERVES: 4

Nutrition Information (Per Serving):
150 Calories / 12g Fat / 9g Carbohydrates / 3g Protein / 500mg Sodium / 4g Sugar

INGREDIENTS:

- 4 medium tomatoes, chopped
- 1 cucumber, sliced
- 1 red onion, thinly sliced
- 1 green bell pepper, sliced
- 1/2 cup Kalamata olives
- 7 oz feta cheese, cut into cubes or crumbled
- 1/4 cup extra virgin olive oil
- 1 tablespoon red wine vinegar
- 1 teaspoon dried oregano
- Salt and pepper to taste

DIRECTIONS:

1. In a large bowl, combine the chopped tomatoes, cucumber slices, red onion slices, green bell pepper slices, and Kalamata olives.
2. Add the cubed or crumbled feta cheese on top of the vegetables.
3. Drizzle the olive oil and red wine vinegar over the salad.
4. Sprinkle with dried oregano, salt, and pepper to taste.
5. Toss the salad gently to combine all the ingredients, ensuring the feta stays somewhat intact.
6. Serve immediately or chill for a few minutes before serving for a more refreshing experience.

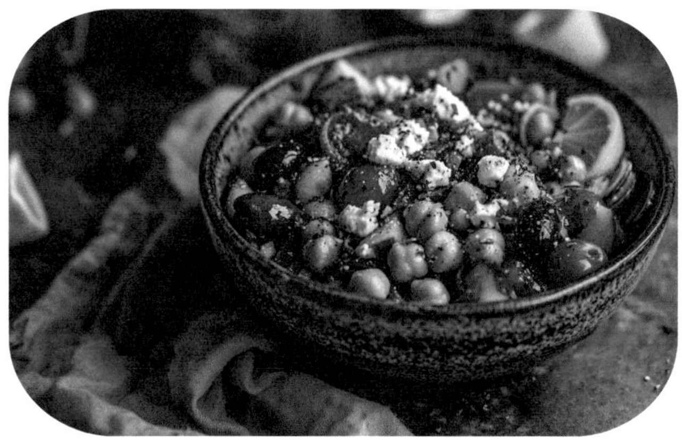

Mediterranean Chickpea Salad

PREPARATION TIME: 15 MINUTES

COOKING TIME: NONE

SERVES: 4

Nutrition Information (Per Serving):
220 Calories / 10g Fat / 25g Carbohydrates / 7g Protein / 400mg Sodium / 4g Sugar

INGREDIENTS:

- 1 can (15 oz) chickpeas, drained and rinsed
- 1 cucumber, diced
- 1 red bell pepper, diced
- 1/2 red onion, finely chopped
- 1/2 cup cherry tomatoes, halved
- 1/4 cup Kalamata olives, sliced
- 1/4 cup feta cheese, crumbled
- 2 tablespoons chopped fresh parsley
- 2 tablespoons extra virgin olive oil
- 1 tablespoon red wine vinegar or lemon juice
- 1 teaspoon dried oregano
- Salt and pepper to taste

DIRECTIONS:

1. In a large bowl, combine the chickpeas, diced cucumber, red bell pepper, red onion, cherry tomatoes, and Kalamata olives.
2. Add the crumbled feta cheese and chopped fresh parsley to the mixture.
3. In a small bowl, whisk together the olive oil, red wine vinegar or lemon juice, dried oregano, salt, and pepper.
4. Pour the dressing over the salad ingredients and toss gently to combine.
5. Taste and adjust seasoning if necessary.
6. Serve immediately or chill in the refrigerator for a more refreshing taste.

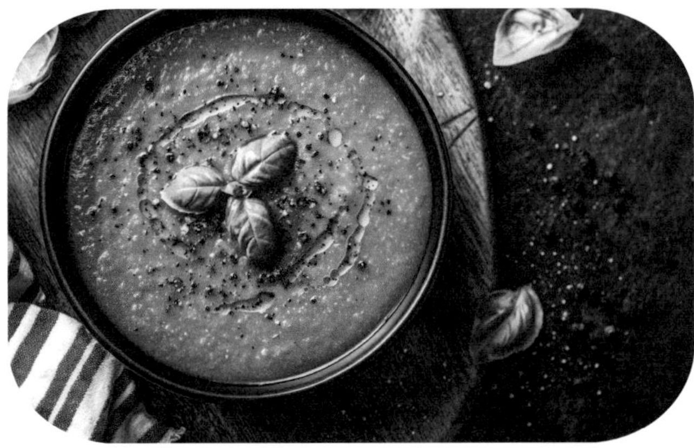

Tomato Basil Soup

 **PREPARATION TIME:** 5 MINUTES

 **COOKING TIME:** 25 MINUTES

SERVES: 4

Nutrition Information (Per Serving):
180 Calories / 9g Fat / 22g Carbohydrates / 4g Protein / 400mg Sodium / 8g Sugar

INGREDIENTS:

- 2 tablespoons olive oil
- 1 onion, chopped
- 3 cloves garlic, minced
- 1 can (28 oz) crushed tomatoes
- 2 cups vegetable broth or water
- 1/2 cup fresh basil leaves, chopped
- 1 teaspoon sugar (optional, to balance acidity)
- Salt and pepper to taste
- 1/4 cup heavy cream or half-and-half (optional, for creamier texture)
- Fresh basil leaves for garnish

DIRECTIONS:

1. In a large pot, heat the olive oil over medium heat.
2. Add the chopped onion and cook for 5-7 minutes until softened.
3. Stir in the minced garlic and cook for another 1-2 minutes until fragrant.
4. Add the crushed tomatoes and vegetable broth or water to the pot. Stir to combine.
5. Bring the soup to a simmer and cook for 15-20 minutes to allow the flavors to meld.
6. Stir in the chopped fresh basil and sugar (if using). Season with salt and pepper to taste.
7. For a creamier texture, stir in the heavy cream or half-and-half just before serving.
8. Use an immersion blender to puree the soup until smooth, or leave it slightly chunky if preferred.
9. Serve the soup hot, garnished with fresh basil leaves.

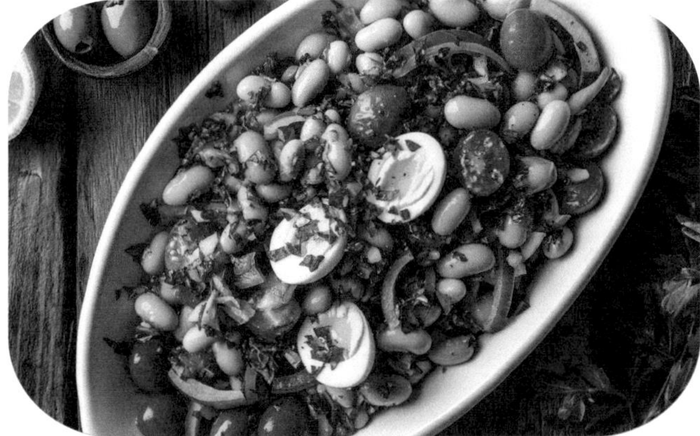

Piyaz (Turkish White Bean Salad)

 **PREPARATION TIME:** 15 MINUTES

 **COOKING TIME:** NONE

 **SERVES:** 4

Nutrition Information (Per Serving):
00 Calories / 10g Fat / 20g Carbohydrates / 6g Protein / 400mg Sodium / 3g Sugar

INGREDIENTS:

- 2 cans (15 oz) white beans, drained
- 1 small red onion, thinly sliced
- 1/2 cup chopped fresh parsley
- 1/2 cup halved cherry tomatoes
- 1/4 cup olive oil
- 2 tbsp red wine vinegar or lemon juice
- 1 tsp sumac (optional)
- Salt and pepper to taste
- 2 hard-boiled eggs, quartered (optional)
- Olives (optional)

DIRECTIONS:

1. In a large bowl, combine the white beans, sliced red onion, chopped parsley, and cherry tomatoes.
2. In a small bowl, whisk together the olive oil, red wine vinegar or lemon juice, sumac (if using), salt, and pepper.
3. Pour the dressing over the bean mixture and toss gently to combine.
4. Taste and adjust seasoning if needed.
5. Garnish with hard-boiled eggs and olives, if desired.
6. Serve immediately or chill for a few minutes before serving.

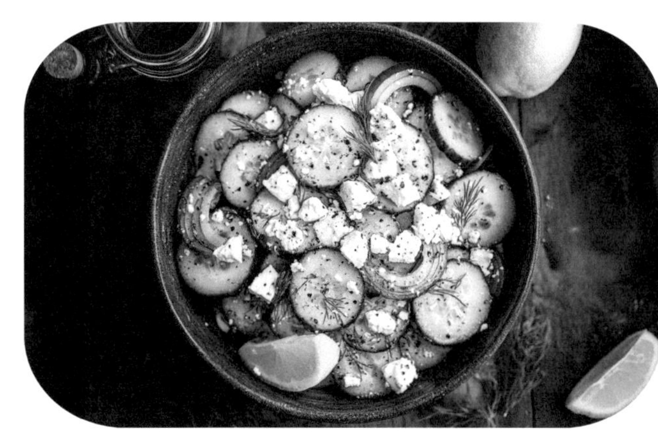

Cucumber Feta Salad

PREPARATION TIME: 10 MINUTES

COOKING TIME: NONE

SERVES: 4

Nutrition Information (Per Serving):
120 Calories / 9g Fat / 7g Carbohydrates / 3g Protein / 350mg Sodium / 3g Sugar

INGREDIENTS:

- 2 large cucumbers, peeled (if preferred) and sliced
- 1/2 cup feta cheese, crumbled
- 1/4 red onion, thinly sliced
- 2 tablespoons extra virgin olive oil
- 1 tablespoon red wine vinegar or lemon juice
- 1 tablespoon chopped fresh dill or mint (optional)
- Salt and pepper to taste

DIRECTIONS:

1. In a large bowl, combine the sliced cucumbers and red onion.
2. Add the crumbled feta cheese to the bowl.
3. Drizzle the olive oil and red wine vinegar or lemon juice over the salad.
4. Add the chopped fresh dill or mint, if using, and season with salt and pepper.
5. Toss gently to combine all ingredients.
6. Serve immediately or chill in the refrigerator for a more refreshing taste.

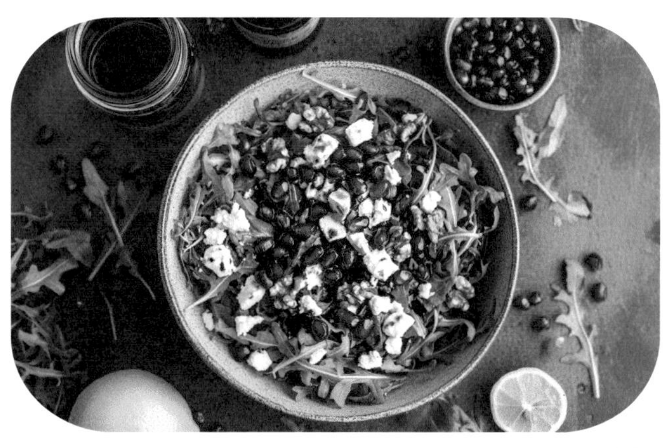

Pomegranate and Arugula Salad

PREPARATION TIME: 10 MINUTES

COOKING TIME: NONE

SERVES: 4

Nutrition Information (Per Serving):
140 Calories / 9g Fat / 9g Carbohydrates / 3g Protein / 220mg Sodium / 6g Sugar

INGREDIENTS:

- 4 cups fresh arugula
- 1/2 cup pomegranate seeds
- 1/4 cup toasted walnuts
- 1/4 cup crumbled feta cheese
- 2 tablespoons olive oil
- 1 tablespoon balsamic vinegar
- Salt and pepper to taste

DIRECTIONS:

1. In a large bowl, combine arugula, pomegranate seeds, walnuts, and crumbled feta cheese.
2. Drizzle with olive oil and balsamic vinegar.
3. Toss gently to coat and season with salt and pepper to taste.
4. Serve immediately for a fresh, crunchy salad.

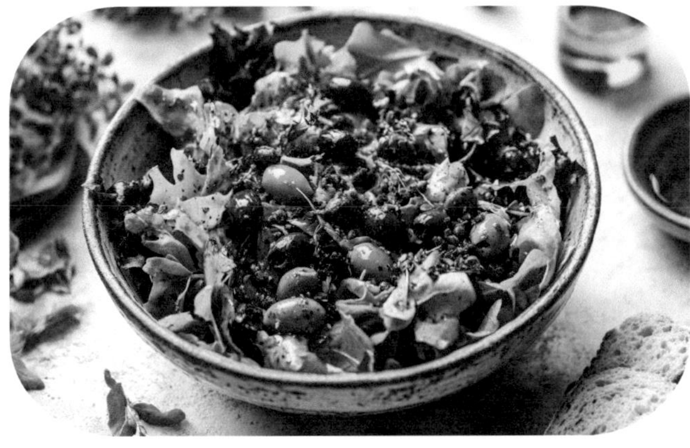

Simple Olive Tapenade Salad

 **PREPARATION TIME:** 10 MINUTES

 **COOKING TIME:** NONE

 **SERVES:** 4

Nutrition Information (Per Serving):
250 Calories / 8g Fat / 35g Carbohydrates / 12g Protein / 450mg Sodium / 5g Sugar

INGREDIENTS:

- 1 cup mixed olives (Kalamata, green, etc.), pitted and chopped
- 1 tablespoon capers, rinsed and chopped
- 1 garlic clove, minced
- 2 tablespoons extra virgin olive oil
- 1 tablespoon lemon juice
- 1 teaspoon chopped fresh thyme or rosemary
- 4 cups mixed salad greens (arugula, spinach, etc.)
- Salt and pepper to taste

DIRECTIONS:

1. In a small bowl, combine the chopped olives, capers, minced garlic, olive oil, lemon juice, and fresh thyme or rosemary. Mix well to create the olive tapenade.
2. Place the mixed salad greens in a large salad bowl.
3. Spoon the olive tapenade over the greens.
4. Toss the salad gently to distribute the tapenade evenly.
5. Season with salt and pepper to taste.
6. Add a few whole olives on top.
7. Serve immediately as a flavorful and savory salad.

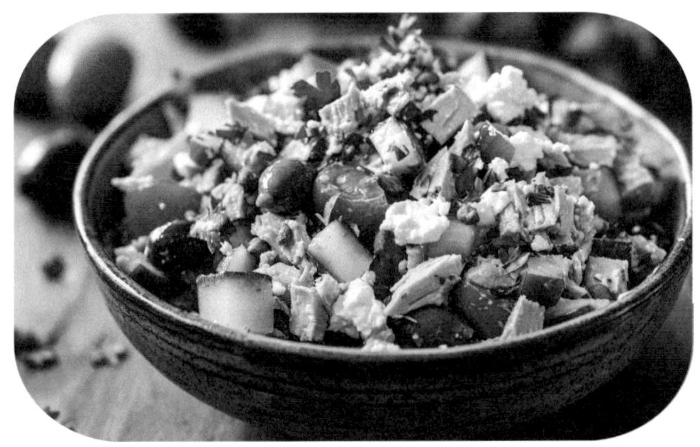

Mediterranean Tuna Salad

 **PREPARATION TIME:** 10 MINUTES

 **COOKING TIME:** NONE

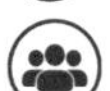 **SERVES:** 4

Nutrition Information (Per Serving):
250 Calories / 15g Fat / 10g Carbohydrates / 22g Protein / 400mg Sodium / 2g Sugar

INGREDIENTS:

- 2 cans (5 oz each) tuna in olive oil, drained
- 1 cup cherry tomatoes, halved
- 1/2 cucumber, diced
- 1/4 red onion, thinly sliced
- 1/4 cup Kalamata olives, halved
- 1/4 cup crumbled feta cheese
- 2 tablespoons capers, drained
- 2 tablespoons fresh parsley, chopped
- 3 tablespoons extra virgin olive oil
- 1 tablespoon lemon juice
- 1 teaspoon dried oregano
- Salt and pepper to taste

DIRECTIONS:

1. In a large bowl, combine the drained tuna, cherry tomatoes, cucumber, red onion, Kalamata olives, feta cheese, capers, and fresh parsley.
2. In a small bowl, whisk together the olive oil, lemon juice, dried oregano, salt, and pepper.
3. Pour the dressing over the salad ingredients and toss gently to combine.
4. Serve the salad immediately or refrigerate for 15-30 minutes to allow the flavors to meld together.

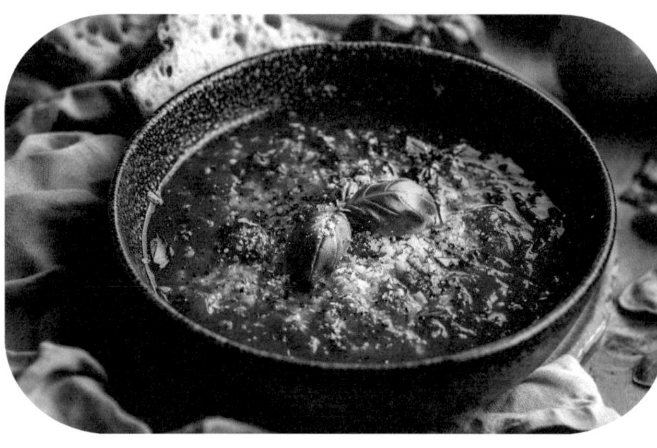

Pappa al Pomodoro (Tomato and Bread Soup)

PREPARATION TIME: 10 MINUTES

COOKING TIME: 20 MINUTES

SERVES: 4

Nutrition Information (Per Serving):
180 Calories / 7g Fat / 25g Carbohydrates / 4g Protein / 500mg Sodium / 5g Sugar

INGREDIENTS:

- 2 tablespoons olive oil
- 1 onion, finely chopped
- 2 garlic cloves, minced
- 4 cups ripe tomatoes, chopped
- 2 cups stale bread, torn into chunks
- 4 cups vegetable broth
- 1/4 cup basil leaves, chopped
- Salt and pepper to taste

DIRECTIONS:

1. Heat olive oil in a pot over medium heat. Sauté onion and garlic until softened.
2. Add chopped tomatoes and cook for 10 minutes until they release their juices.
3. Stir in bread chunks and vegetable broth. Simmer for 10 minutes, stirring occasionally.
4. Add chopped basil and season with salt and pepper.
5. Serve warm with an extra drizzle of olive oil if desired.

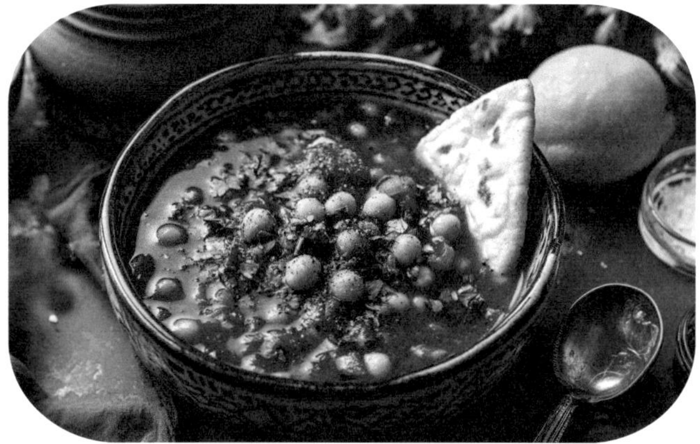

Moroccan Harira Soup

PREPARATION TIME: 10 MINUTES

COOKING TIME: 20 MINUTES

SERVES: 4

Nutrition Information (Per Serving):
200 Calories / 8g Fat / 28g Carbohydrates / 7g Protein / 400mg Sodium / 4g Sugar

INGREDIENTS:

- 1 tbsp olive oil
- 1 onion, chopped
- 2 garlic cloves, minced
- 1 tsp turmeric,1 tsp cinnamon, 1 tsp paprika, 1/2 tsp cumin
- 1 can (15 oz) chickpeas, drained
- 1/2 cup cooked lentils (or canned, drained)
- 4 cups vegetable broth
- 2 tbsp tomato paste
- 1 tomato, grated
- 1/4 cup parsley, chopped (optional)
- Juice of 1/2 lemon
- Salt and pepper

DIRECTIONS:

1. In a large pot, heat olive oil over medium heat.
2. Add the chopped onion and minced garlic to the pot. Sauté for 3-4 minutes until the onion becomes translucent and the garlic is fragrant.
3. Stir in the ground turmeric, cinnamon, paprika, and cumin. Cook for 1 minute to toast the spices and release their aroma.
4. Mix in the grated tomato and tomato paste. Stir well and cook for 2-3 minutes to allow the tomato to soften and blend with the spices.
5. Add the vegetable broth to the pot and bring to a gentle boil.
6. Add the cooked lentils and chickpeas to the pot. Stir everything together and simmer for 10 minutes to let the flavors meld.
7. Add salt, pepper, and lemon juice to taste. Stir in the fresh parsley (if using).
8. If the soup is too thick, add a bit more broth or water until the desired consistency is reached. Simmer for an additional 2-3 minutes.
9. Ladle the soup into bowls and serve hot. For an authentic touch, serve with warm flatbread or a wedge of lemon on the side.

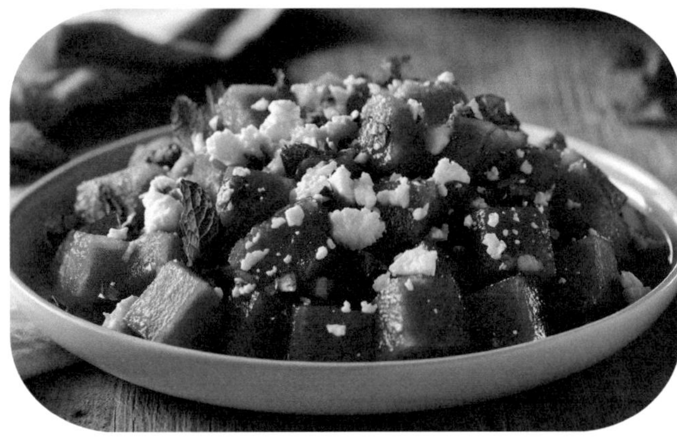

Watermelon and Feta Salad

 **PREPARATION TIME:** 10 MINUTES

 **COOKING TIME:** NONE

 **SERVES:** 4

Nutrition Information (Per Serving):
150 Calories / 8g Fat / 18g Carbohydrates / 4g Protein / 250mg Sodium / 14g Sugar

INGREDIENTS:

- 4 cups watermelon, cubed
- 1 cup feta cheese, crumbled
- 1/4 cup fresh mint leaves, chopped
- 2 tablespoons olive oil
- 1 tablespoon balsamic glaze or balsamic vinegar
- Salt and pepper to taste

DIRECTIONS:

1. In a large bowl, combine the watermelon cubes, crumbled feta, and chopped mint.
2. Drizzle with olive oil and balsamic glaze or vinegar.
3. Toss gently to combine.
4. Season with salt and pepper to taste.
5. Serve immediately and enjoy a refreshing and flavorful salad.

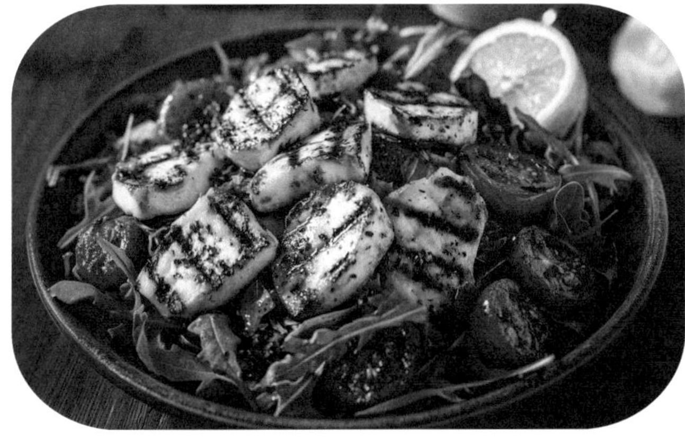

Grilled Halloumi Salad

 **PREPARATION TIME:** 10 MINUTES

 **COOKING TIME:** 10 MINUTES

 **SERVES:** 4

Nutrition Information (Per Serving):
350 Calories / 28g Fat / 12g Carbohydrates / 18g Protein / 450mg Sodium / 4g Sugar

INGREDIENTS:

- 2 blocks (about 7 oz each) halloumi cheese, sliced
- 4 cups mixed salad greens (arugula, spinach, or your choice)
- 1 cup cherry tomatoes, halved
- 4 tablespoons olive oil
- 2 tablespoons fresh lemon juice
- 1 teaspoon dried oregano (optional)
- Salt and pepper, to taste

DIRECTIONS:

1. Heat a grill pan or outdoor grill over medium heat. Grill the halloumi slices for 2-3 minutes on each side until golden and grill marks appear.
2. In a large salad bowl, combine the mixed greens and cherry tomatoes. Top with the grilled halloumi.
3. In a small bowl, whisk together olive oil, lemon juice, oregano (if using), and a pinch of salt and pepper.
4. Drizzle the dressing over the salad and toss gently to combine. Serve immediately while the halloumi is still warm.

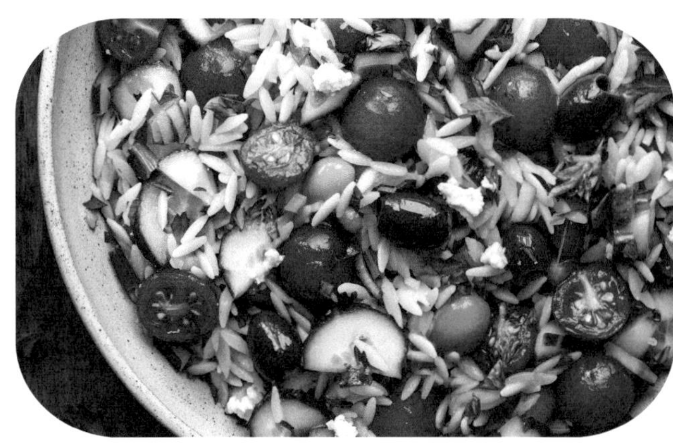

Simple Orzo Pasta Salad

PREPARATION TIME: 10 MINUTES

COOKING TIME: 10 MINUTES

SERVES: 4

Nutrition Information (Per Serving):
220 Calories / 8g Fat / 30g Carbohydrates / 6g Protein / 350mg Sodium / 2g Sugar

INGREDIENTS:

- 1 cup orzo pasta
- 1/2 cup cherry tomatoes, halved
- 1/2 cucumber, diced
- 1/4 cup red onion, finely chopped
- 1/4 cup Kalamata olives, sliced
- 1/4 cup feta cheese, crumbled
- 2 tablespoons fresh parsley, chopped
- 2 tablespoons olive oil
- 1 tablespoon lemon juice
- Salt and pepper to taste

DIRECTIONS:

1. Bring a large pot of salted water to a boil. Add the orzo and cook according to package instructions, about 8-10 minutes. Drain and rinse under cold water to cool.
2. In a large bowl, combine the halved cherry tomatoes, diced cucumber, chopped red onion, sliced Kalamata olives, and crumbled feta cheese.
3. Add the cooked orzo to the bowl with the vegetables. Drizzle with olive oil and lemon juice.
4. Season with salt and pepper to taste. Toss gently to combine all the ingredients.
5. Serve the salad chilled or at room temperature, garnished with chopped fresh parsley.

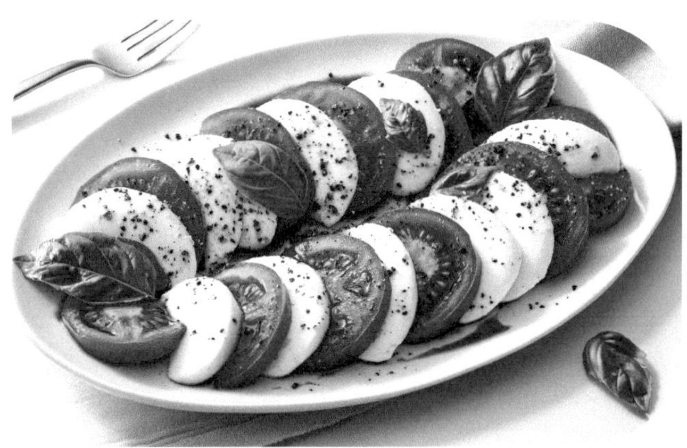

Caprese Salad

PREPARATION TIME: 10 MINUTES

COOKING TIME: NONE

SERVES: 4

Nutrition Information (Per Serving):
200 Calories / 16g Fat / 6g Carbohydrates / 7g Protein / 150mg Sodium / 4g Sugar

INGREDIENTS:

- 3-4 large ripe tomatoes, sliced
- 1 pound fresh mozzarella cheese, sliced
- 1/4 cup fresh basil leaves
- 2 tablespoons extra virgin olive oil
- 1 tablespoon balsamic glaze (optional)
- Salt and pepper to taste

DIRECTIONS:

1. Arrange the tomato slices and mozzarella slices alternately on a large platter, slightly overlapping them.
2. Tuck fresh basil leaves between the tomato and mozzarella slices.
3. Drizzle the salad with extra virgin olive oil, and balsamic glaze if using.
4. Season with salt and pepper to taste.
5. Serve the salad immediately, as a refreshing and elegant side dish.

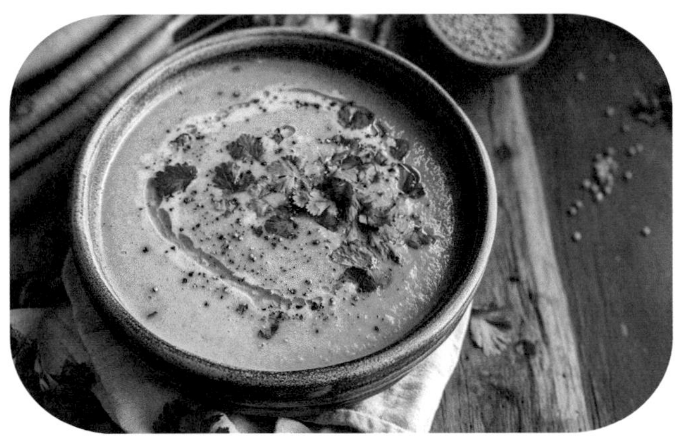

Carrot and Cumin Soup

 **PREPARATION TIME:** 5 MINUTES

 **COOKING TIME:** 25 MINUTES

 **SERVES:** 4

Nutrition Information (Per Serving):
150 Calories / 7g Fat / 20g Carbohydrates / 2g Protein / 300mg Sodium / 8g Sugar

INGREDIENTS:

- 2 tablespoons olive oil
- 1 onion, chopped
- 2 garlic cloves, minced
- 1 teaspoon ground cumin
- 1 pound carrots, peeled and sliced
- 4 cups vegetable broth
- Salt and pepper to taste
- Fresh cilantro or parsley for garnish (optional)
- A squeeze of lemon juice (optional)

DIRECTIONS:

1. In a large pot, heat olive oil over medium heat. Add the chopped onion and sauté for 5-7 minutes until softened. Add the minced garlic and cumin, and cook for another 1-2 minutes until fragrant.
2. Add the sliced carrots to the pot and pour in the vegetable broth. Bring to a boil, then reduce the heat and simmer for about 20 minutes, until the carrots are tender.
3. Use an immersion blender to puree the soup until smooth, or transfer the soup to a blender and blend in batches. Return the soup to the pot.
4. Season with salt and pepper to taste. If desired, add a squeeze of lemon juice for extra brightness.
5. Serve the soup hot, garnished with fresh cilantro or parsley

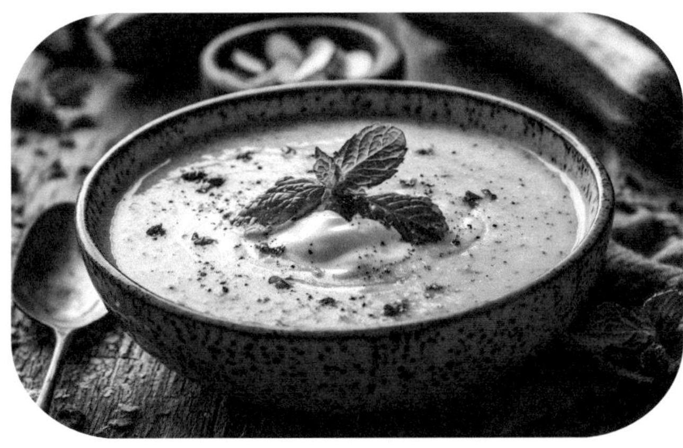

Zucchini and Mint Soup

 **PREPARATION TIME:** 10 MINUTES

 **COOKING TIME:** 20 MINUTES

 **SERVES:** 4

Nutrition Information (Per Serving):
120 Calories / 6g Fat / 12g Carbohydrates / 3g Protein / 250mg Sodium / 4g Sugar

INGREDIENTS:

- 2 tablespoons olive oil
- 1 onion, chopped
- 2 garlic cloves, minced
- 4 medium zucchinis, sliced
- 4 cups vegetable broth
- 1/4 cup fresh mint leaves, chopped
- Salt and pepper to taste
- Greek yogurt or sour cream for garnish (optional)

DIRECTIONS:

1. In a large pot, heat olive oil over medium heat. Add the chopped onion and sauté for 5-7 minutes until softened. Add the minced garlic and cook for another 1-2 minutes until fragrant.
2. Add the sliced zucchini to the pot and pour in the vegetable broth. Bring to a boil, then reduce the heat and simmer for about 15 minutes, until the zucchini is tender.
3. Use an immersion blender to puree the soup until smooth, or transfer the soup to a blender and blend in batches. Return the soup to the pot.
4. Stir in the chopped fresh mint and season with salt and pepper to taste.
5. Serve the soup hot, garnished with a dollop of Greek yogurt or sour cream if desired.

Chapter 4

VEGGIES and SIDE DISHES

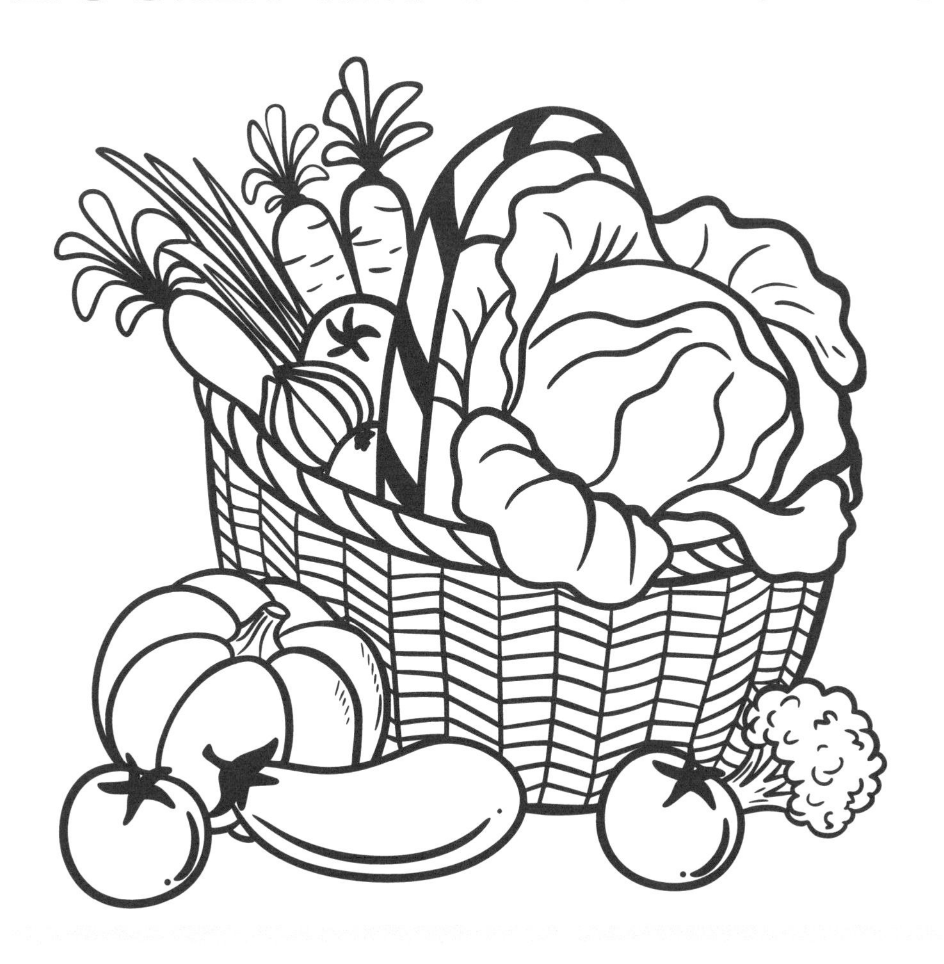

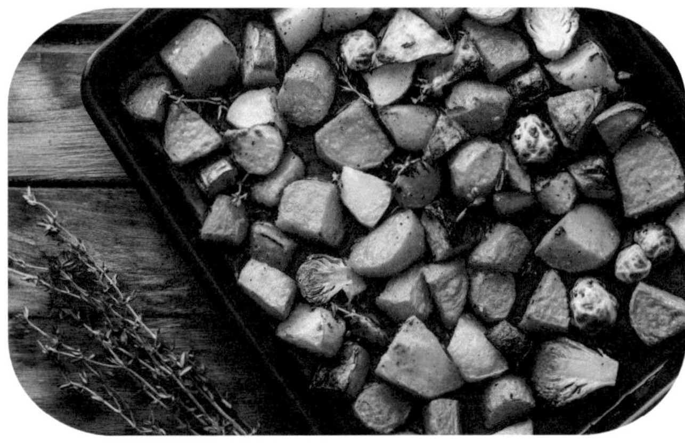

Honey and Thyme Roasted Vegetables

PREPARATION TIME: 5 MINUTES

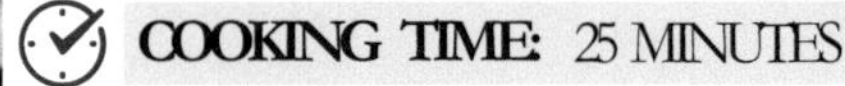

COOKING TIME: 25 MINUTES

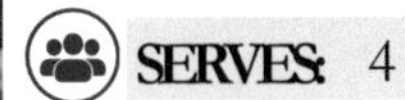

SERVES: 4

Nutrition Information (Per Serving):
180 Calories / 9g Fat / 25g Carbohydrates / 3g Protein / 250mg Sodium / 10g Sugar

INGREDIENTS:

- 4 cups mixed vegetables (such as carrots, parsnips, sweet potatoes, and Brussels sprouts), cut into bite-sized pieces
- 2 tablespoons olive oil
- 2 tablespoons honey
- 1 tablespoon fresh thyme leaves (or 1 teaspoon dried thyme)
- Salt and pepper to taste
- 1 tablespoon balsamic vinegar (optional, for added flavor)

DIRECTIONS:

1. Preheat your oven to 400°F (200°C).
2. In a large bowl, combine the mixed vegetables, olive oil, honey, thyme, salt, and pepper. Toss until the vegetables are evenly coated.
3. Spread the vegetables in a single layer on a baking sheet lined with parchment paper.
4. Roast in the preheated oven for 25-30 minutes, or until the vegetables are tender and caramelized, stirring halfway through for even cooking.
5. If using, drizzle the roasted vegetables with balsamic vinegar and toss gently to combine.
6. Serve hot, as a delicious and flavorful side dish.

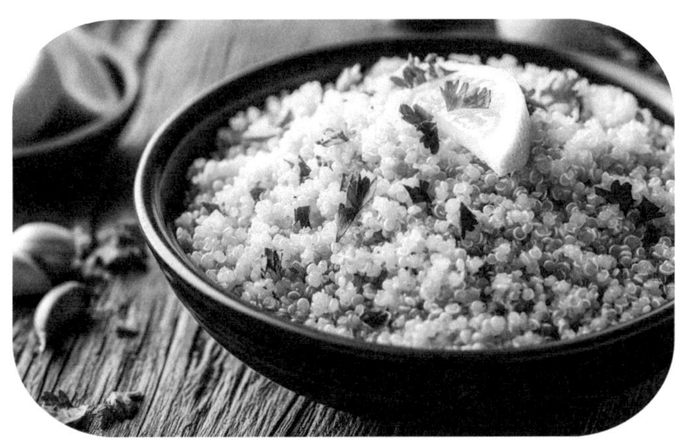

Lemon Garlic Quinoa

PREPARATION TIME: 5 MINUTES

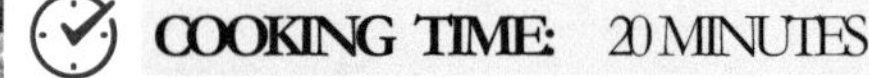

COOKING TIME: 20 MINUTES

SERVES: 4

Nutrition Information (Per Serving):
160 Calories / 6g Fat / 24g Carbohydrates / 5g Protein / 150mg Sodium / 1g Sugar

INGREDIENTS:

- 1 cup quinoa, rinsed
- 2 cups vegetable broth or water
- 2 tablespoons olive oil
- 2 cloves garlic, minced
- Zest and juice of 1 lemon
- Salt and pepper to taste
- 2 tablespoons fresh parsley, chopped (optional, for garnish)

DIRECTIONS:

1. In a medium saucepan, combine the rinsed quinoa and vegetable broth or water. Bring to a boil over medium-high heat.
2. Reduce the heat to low, cover, and simmer for about 15 minutes, or until the quinoa is cooked and the liquid is absorbed. Remove from heat and let it sit, covered, for 5 minutes.
3. While the quinoa is cooking, heat the olive oil in a small skillet over medium heat. Add the minced garlic and sauté for 1-2 minutes until fragrant, being careful not to burn it.
4. Fluff the cooked quinoa with a fork and transfer it to a large bowl. Add the sautéed garlic, lemon zest, and lemon juice. Stir to combine.
5. Season with salt and pepper to taste.
6. Serve warm, garnished with chopped fresh parsley if desired.

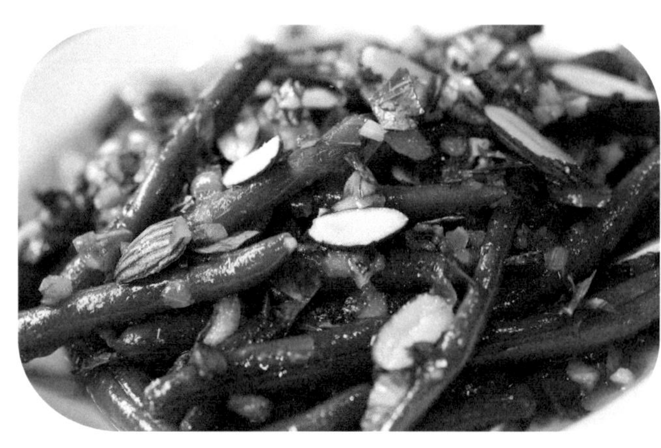

Turkish Green Beans with Almonds

PREPARATION TIME: 5 MINUTES

COOKING TIME: 25 MINUTES

SERVES: 4

Nutrition Information (Per Serving):
130 Calories / 8g Fat / 12g Carbohydrates / 3g Protein / 200mg Sodium / 3g Sugar

INGREDIENTS:

- 1 pound green beans, trimmed
- 2 tablespoons olive oil
- 1 small onion, finely chopped
- 3 cloves garlic, minced
- 1 large tomato, chopped
- 1/4 cup sliced almonds
- 1/2 teaspoon ground cumin
- Salt and pepper to taste
- Juice of 1/2 lemon
- Fresh parsley, chopped (optional, for garnish)

DIRECTIONS:

1. Heat olive oil in a large skillet over medium heat. Sauté the onion for 3-4 minutes until softened, then add garlic and cook for 1-2 minutes until fragrant.
2. Add the chopped tomato and cook for 5 minutes to create a sauce.
3. Stir in the green beans, cover, and cook for 15-20 minutes, stirring occasionally, until tender.
4. Toast the almonds in a small pan over medium heat for 2-3 minutes until golden.
5. Season the green beans with cumin, salt, and pepper. Drizzle with lemon juice, stir, and transfer to a serving dish.
6. Top with toasted almonds and garnish with fresh parsley if desired.

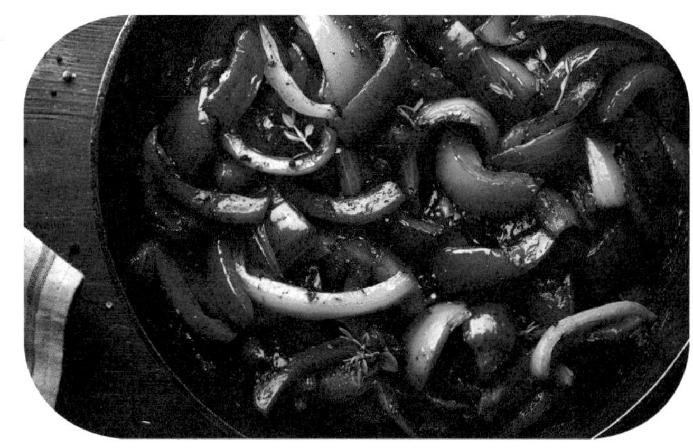

Caramelized Onions and Peppers

PREPARATION TIME: 10 MINUTES

COOKING TIME: 25 MINUTES

SERVES: 4

Nutrition Information (Per Serving):
150 Calories / 7g Fat / 20g Carbohydrates / 2g Protein / 200mg Sodium / 8g Sugar

INGREDIENTS:

- 2 large onions, thinly sliced
- 2 large bell peppers (any color), thinly sliced
- 2 tablespoons olive oil
- 1 tablespoon balsamic vinegar (optional)
- 1 teaspoon sugar (optional, for extra caramelization)
- Salt and pepper to taste
- Fresh thyme or basil for garnish (optional)

DIRECTIONS:

1. In a large skillet, heat the olive oil over medium heat.
2. Add the sliced onions to the skillet and cook, stirring occasionally, for about 10 minutes until the onions begin to soften and turn golden.
3. Add the sliced bell peppers to the skillet. Continue to cook, stirring occasionally, for another 15-20 minutes, until both the onions and peppers are deeply caramelized and tender.
4. If desired, stir in the balsamic vinegar and sugar for extra depth of flavor and enhanced caramelization. Cook for an additional 2-3 minutes.
5. Season with salt and pepper to taste.
6. Garnish with fresh thyme or basil if desired, and serve warm.

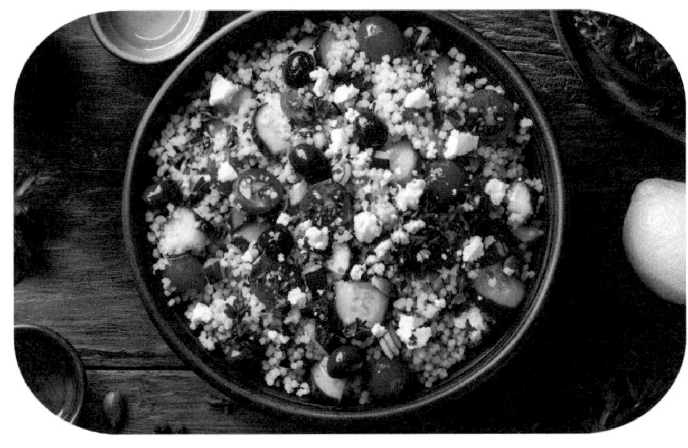

Mediterranean Couscous

PREPARATION TIME: 10 MINUTES

COOKING TIME: 15 MINUTES

SERVES: 4

Nutrition Information (Per Serving):
210 Calories / 7g Fat / 32g Carbohydrates / 6g Protein / 300mg Sodium / 2g Sugar

INGREDIENTS:

- 1 cup couscous
- 1 1/4 cups vegetable broth or water
- 2 tablespoons olive oil
- 1/2 cup cherry tomatoes, halved
- 1/2 cup cucumber, diced
- 1/4 cup Kalamata olives, sliced
- 1/4 cup red onion, finely chopped
- 1/4 cup crumbled feta cheese
- 2 tablespoons fresh parsley, chopped
- Juice of 1 lemon
- Salt and pepper to taste

DIRECTIONS:

1. In a medium saucepan, bring the vegetable broth or water to a boil. Stir in the couscous, cover, and remove from heat. Let it sit for 5 minutes, then fluff with a fork.
2. In a large bowl, combine the couscous with the cherry tomatoes, cucumber, Kalamata olives, red onion, and crumbled feta cheese.
3. Drizzle the olive oil and lemon juice over the couscous mixture. Toss to combine.
4. Season with salt and pepper to taste.
5. Garnish with fresh parsley and serve the couscous at room temperature or slightly chilled.

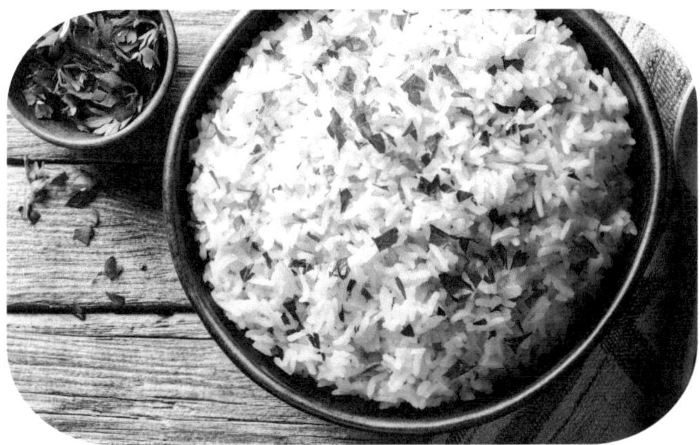

Simple Greek Rice Pilaf

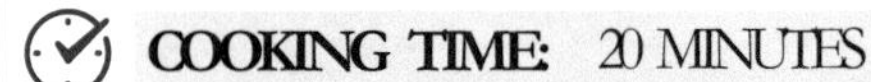

PREPARATION TIME: 5 MINUTES

COOKING TIME: 20 MINUTES

SERVES: 4

Nutrition Information (Per Serving):
180 Calories / 5g Fat / 30g Carbohydrates / 4g Protein / 300mg Sodium / 1g Sugar

INGREDIENTS:

- 1 cup long-grain rice (like basmati or jasmine)
- 2 cups vegetable broth or water
- 1 small onion, finely chopped
- 2 tablespoons olive oil
- 1 garlic clove, minced
- 1/4 teaspoon ground cinnamon (optional)
- 1/4 teaspoon ground allspice (optional)
- Salt and pepper to taste
- 2 tablespoons fresh parsley, chopped (for garnish)
- 1 tablespoon fresh lemon juice (optional, for a fresh zing)

DIRECTIONS:

1. In a large saucepan, heat the olive oil over medium heat. Add the chopped onion and sauté for about 3-4 minutes until softened.
2. Add the minced garlic and cook for another 1-2 minutes until fragrant.
3. Stir in the rice, coating it well with the olive oil, and cook for 2 minutes, allowing it to lightly toast.
4. Add the vegetable broth, cinnamon, and allspice (if using). Bring the mixture to a boil, then reduce the heat to low, cover, and simmer for about 15 minutes, or until the rice is cooked and the liquid is absorbed.
5. Remove the pan from heat and let it sit, covered, for 5 minutes. Fluff the rice with a fork.
6. Season with salt and pepper to taste, and stir in the fresh lemon juice, if using.
7. Garnish with chopped fresh parsley before serving.

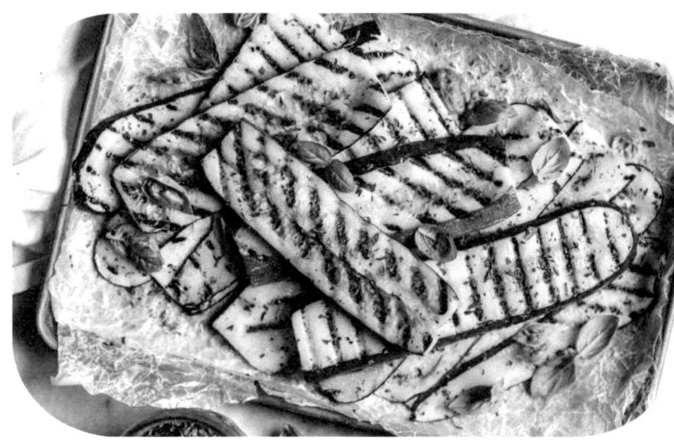

Grilled Zucchini

PREPARATION TIME: 5 MINUTES

COOKING TIME: 10 MINUTES

SERVES: 4

Nutrition Information (Per Serving):
70 Calories / 5g Fat / 6g Carbohydrates / 1g Protein / 150mg Sodium / 3g Sugar

INGREDIENTS:

- 4 medium zucchinis, sliced lengthwise into 1/4-inch thick strips
- 2 tablespoons olive oil
- 1 teaspoon garlic powder or 2 cloves fresh garlic, minced
- Salt and pepper to taste
- 1 tablespoon fresh lemon juice (optional)
- 1 tablespoon fresh parsley or basil, chopped (for garnish)

DIRECTIONS:

1. Preheat your grill to medium-high heat.
2. In a large bowl, toss the zucchini slices with olive oil, garlic powder (or minced fresh garlic), salt, and pepper until evenly coated.
3. Place the zucchini slices on the grill and cook for 3-4 minutes on each side, until grill marks appear and the zucchini is tender but not mushy.
4. Remove the zucchini from the grill and drizzle with fresh lemon juice, if desired.
5. Garnish with chopped fresh parsley or basil before serving.

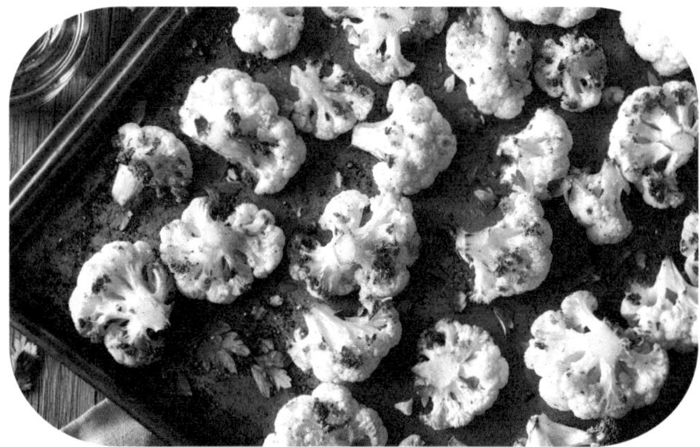

Garlic Roasted Cauliflower

PREPARATION TIME: 5 MINUTES

COOKING TIME: 25 MINUTES

SERVES: 4

Nutrition Information (Per Serving):
120 Calories / 7g Fat / 12g Carbohydrates / 3g Protein / 200mg Sodium / 2g Sugar

INGREDIENTS:

- 1 large head of cauliflower, cut into florets
- 3 cloves garlic, minced
- 3 tablespoons olive oil
- 1 teaspoon smoked paprika (optional)
- Salt and pepper to taste
- 1 tablespoon fresh parsley, chopped (optional, for garnish)
- 1 tablespoon lemon juice (optional, for garnish)

DIRECTIONS:

1. Preheat your oven to 400°F (200°C).
2. In a large bowl, toss the cauliflower florets with olive oil, minced garlic, smoked paprika (if using), salt, and pepper until evenly coated.
3. Spread the cauliflower in a single layer on a baking sheet lined with parchment paper.
4. Roast in the preheated oven for 20-25 minutes, stirring halfway through, until the cauliflower is tender and golden brown.
5. Remove from the oven and drizzle with lemon juice, if desired. Garnish with chopped fresh parsley.

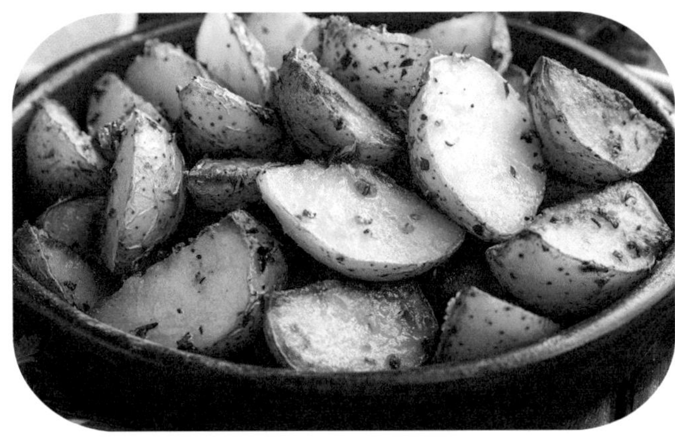

Herb-Roasted Potatoes with Olive Oil

PREPARATION TIME: 5 MINUTES

COOKING TIME: 20-25 MINUTES

SERVES: 4

Nutrition Information (Per Serving):
210 Calories / 9g Fat / 30g Carbohydrates / 3g Protein / 300mg Sodium / 1g Sugar

INGREDIENTS:

- 1 lb baby potatoes, halved or quartered
- 2 tablespoons olive oil
- 1 teaspoon dried oregano
- 1 teaspoon dried thyme
- 1/2 teaspoon garlic powder
- 1/4 teaspoon smoked paprika
- Salt and pepper to taste
- 1 tablespoon fresh parsley, chopped (for garnish)

DIRECTIONS:

1. Place halved or quartered potatoes in a pot of salted boiling water. Cook for 3-5 minutes until slightly tender, then drain.
2. While potatoes boil, preheat the oven to 425°F (220°C) and line a baking sheet with parchment paper.
3. Toss the drained potatoes in a bowl with olive oil, oregano, thyme, garlic powder, smoked paprika, salt, and pepper.
4. Spread the seasoned potatoes on the baking sheet in a single layer, cut-side down, and bake for 15-20 minutes, flipping halfway through, until golden and crispy.
5. Sprinkle with fresh parsley and serve warm as a side dish.

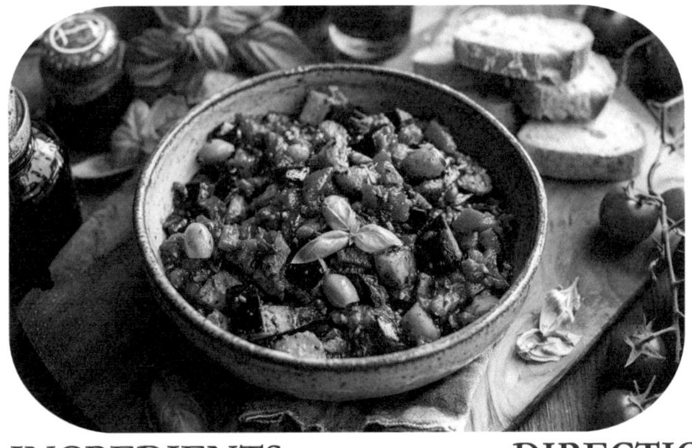

Eggplant Caponata

PREPARATION TIME: 10 MINUTES

COOKING TIME: 20 MINUTES

SERVES: 4

Nutrition Information (Per Serving):
180 Calories / 10g Fat / 20g Carbohydrates / 3g Protein / 350mg Sodium / 8g Sugar

INGREDIENTS:

- 1 large eggplant, diced
- 2 tablespoons olive oil
- 1 small onion, chopped
- 2 garlic cloves, minced
- 1 red bell pepper, diced
- 1 can (14 oz) diced tomatoes
- 2 tablespoons capers, rinsed
- 2 tablespoons red wine vinegar
- 1 tablespoon sugar
- 1/4 cup Kalamata olives, sliced
- Salt and pepper to taste
- Fresh basil leaves for garnish

DIRECTIONS:

1. Heat olive oil in a large skillet over medium heat. Sauté the eggplant for 5-7 minutes until softened.
2. Add onion, garlic, and red bell pepper. Cook for another 3-4 minutes until the vegetables are softened.
3. Stir in the diced tomatoes, capers, red wine vinegar, sugar, and olives. Season with salt and pepper.
4. Simmer uncovered for 10 minutes, stirring occasionally, until the mixture thickens and flavors meld.
5. Garnish with fresh basil leaves and serve warm or at room temperature as a side dish or topping for crusty bread.

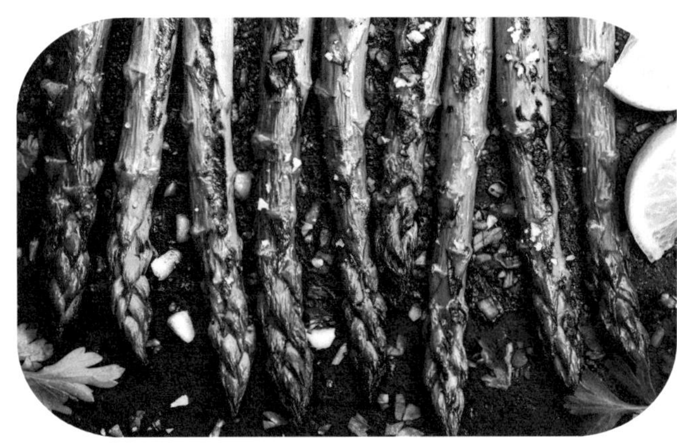

Grilled Asparagus with Lemon

PREPARATION TIME: 5 MINUTES

COOKING TIME: 10 MINUTES

SERVES: 4

Nutrition Information (Per Serving):
80 Calories / 7g Fat / 5g Carbohydrates / 2g Protein / 150mg Sodium / 2g Sugar

INGREDIENTS:

- 1 bunch of asparagus, trimmed
- 2 tablespoons olive oil
- 1 lemon (zested and juiced)
- 2 cloves garlic, minced
- Salt and pepper to taste
- 1 tablespoon grated Parmesan cheese (optional)
- Fresh parsley, chopped (optional, for garnish)

DIRECTIONS:

1. Preheat your grill to medium-high heat.
2. In a large bowl, toss the asparagus with olive oil, minced garlic, lemon zest, salt, and pepper until evenly coated.
3. Place the asparagus on the grill in a single layer and cook for 3-4 minutes on each side, until tender and slightly charred.
4. Remove the asparagus from the grill and drizzle with fresh lemon juice.
5. If desired, sprinkle with grated Parmesan cheese and garnish with chopped fresh parsley before serving.

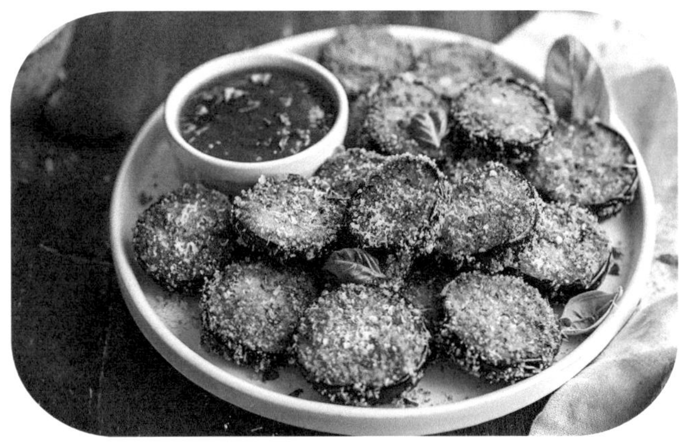

Crispy Eggplant Rounds

PREPARATION TIME: 10 MINUTES

COOKING TIME: 20 MINUTES

SERVES: 4

Nutrition Information (Per Serving):
200 Calories / 10g Fat / 20g Carbohydrates / 4g Protein / 350mg Sodium / 2g Sugar

INGREDIENTS:

- 1 large eggplant, sliced into 1/4-inch rounds
- 1 cup breadcrumbs
- 1/2 cup grated Parmesan cheese
- 1 teaspoon dried oregano
- 1/2 teaspoon garlic powder
- 2 large eggs, beaten
- Olive oil for brushing or spraying
- Salt and pepper to taste

DIRECTIONS:

1. Preheat the oven to 425°F (220°C) and line a baking sheet with parchment paper.
2. Lightly salt the eggplant slices and let them rest for 5 minutes. Pat them dry with a paper towel.
3. In one bowl, combine breadcrumbs, Parmesan cheese, oregano, and garlic powder. In another bowl, beat the eggs.
4. Dip each eggplant slice into the egg mixture, then coat it in the breadcrumb mixture, pressing gently to adhere.
5. Arrange the coated slices on the baking sheet in a single layer. Lightly brush or spray with olive oil.
6. Bake for 15-20 minutes, flipping halfway through, until golden brown and crispy.
7. Serve warm as a snack, appetizer, or side dish. Pair with marinara sauce or tzatziki for dipping.

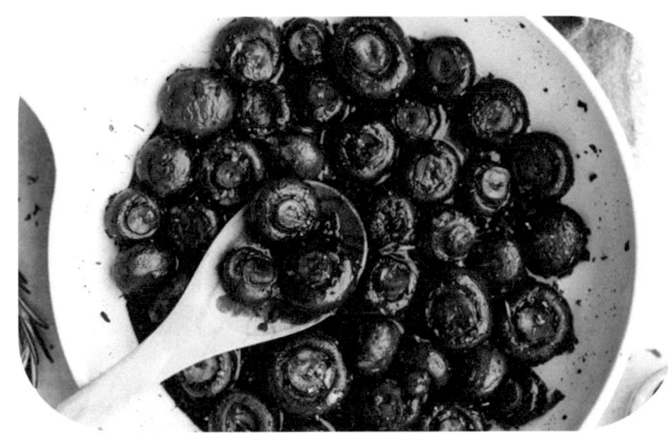

Balsamic Glazed Mushrooms

 **PREPARATION TIME:** 10 MINUTES

 **COOKING TIME:** 15 MINUTES

 **SERVES:** 4

Nutrition Information (Per Serving):
110 Calories / 7g Fat / 9g Carbohydrates / 2g Protein / 250mg Sodium / 4g Sugar

INGREDIENTS:

- 1 lb cremini or button mushrooms, cleaned and halved
- 2 tablespoons olive oil
- 2 garlic cloves, minced
- 2 tablespoons balsamic vinegar
- 1 teaspoon honey or maple syrup
- 1 teaspoon fresh thyme leaves (or 1/2 teaspoon dried thyme)
- Salt and pepper to taste

DIRECTIONS:

1. Heat olive oil in a large skillet over medium heat.
2. Add the mushrooms and cook for 5-7 minutes, stirring occasionally, until they release their moisture and start to brown.
3. Stir in the garlic and thyme, cooking for 1 minute until fragrant.
4. Drizzle the balsamic vinegar and honey (or maple syrup) over the mushrooms. Stir well to coat evenly.
5. Cook for an additional 3-5 minutes, letting the glaze thicken and caramelize slightly.
6. Season with salt and pepper to taste. Serve warm as a side dish or topping for salads, pasta, or toast.

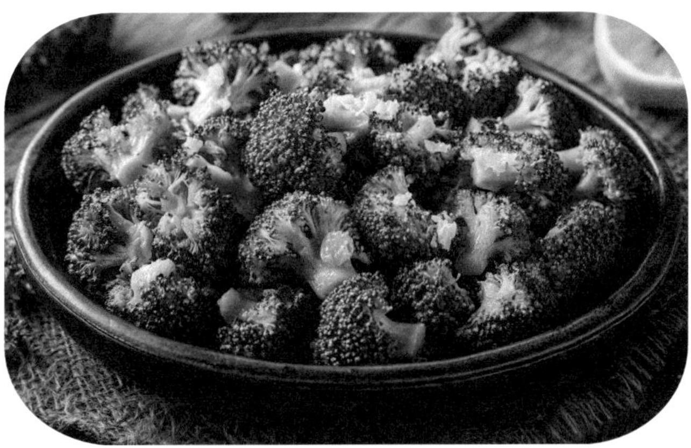

Broccoli with Lemon and Garlic

 **PREPARATION TIME:** 5 MINUTES

 **COOKING TIME:** 10 MINUTES

 **SERVES:** 4

Nutrition Information (Per Serving):
90 Calories / 6g Fat / 9g Carbohydrates / 3g Protein / 120mg Sodium / 2g Sugar

INGREDIENTS:

- 1 large head of broccoli, cut into florets
- 2 tablespoons olive oil
- 3 cloves garlic, minced
- Zest and juice of 1 lemon
- Salt and pepper to taste
- Red pepper flakes (optional, for a bit of heat)
- Fresh parsley, chopped (optional, for garnish)

DIRECTIONS:

1. Steam the broccoli florets in a steamer basket over boiling water for 4-5 minutes, until just tender but still crisp.
2. While the broccoli is steaming, heat olive oil in a large skillet over medium heat. Add the minced garlic and sauté for 1-2 minutes until fragrant.
3. Add the steamed broccoli to the skillet and toss to coat in the garlic and olive oil. Cook for 2-3 minutes, stirring occasionally.
4. Remove from heat and add the lemon zest and juice. Season with salt, pepper, and red pepper flakes if using. Toss to combine.
5. Transfer to a serving dish and garnish with fresh parsley if desired.

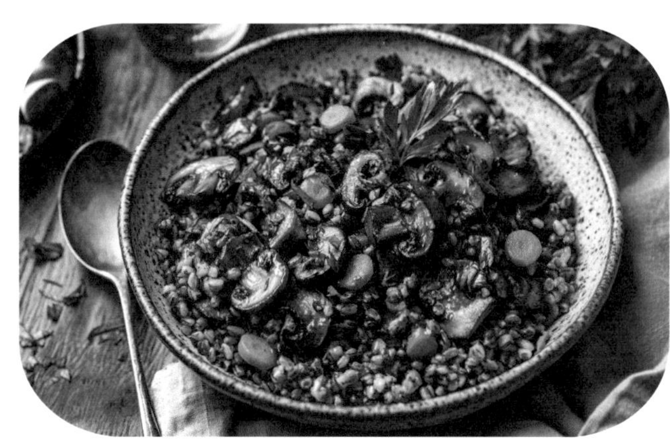

Farro with Mushrooms and Carrots

PREPARATION TIME: 5 MINUTES

COOKING TIME: 25 MINUTES

SERVES: 4

Nutrition Information (Per Serving):
220 Calories / 7g Fat / 35g Carbohydrates / 6g Protein / 300mg Sodium / 4g Sugar

INGREDIENTS:

- 1 cup farro, rinsed
- 2 cups vegetable broth (or water)
- 2 tablespoons olive oil
- 1 medium onion, chopped
- 2 garlic cloves, minced
- 1 lb mushrooms, sliced
- 2 medium carrots, diced
- 1 teaspoon dried thyme
- Salt and pepper to taste
- 2 tablespoons fresh parsley, chopped (for garnish)

DIRECTIONS:

1. In a medium pot, combine farro and vegetable broth. Bring to a boil, reduce heat, cover, and simmer for 15-20 minutes until tender. Drain any excess liquid.
2. While farro cooks, heat olive oil in a large skillet over medium heat.
3. Add the onion and garlic to the skillet. Sauté for 2-3 minutes until softened.
4. Stir in the mushrooms and carrots, cooking for 5-7 minutes until mushrooms release their moisture and carrots are tender.
5. Add thyme, salt, and pepper. Stir to combine.
6. Toss the cooked farro into the skillet with the mushroom and carrot mixture. Stir well to coat and heat through.
7. Garnish with fresh parsley and serve warm as a hearty side dish or main meal.

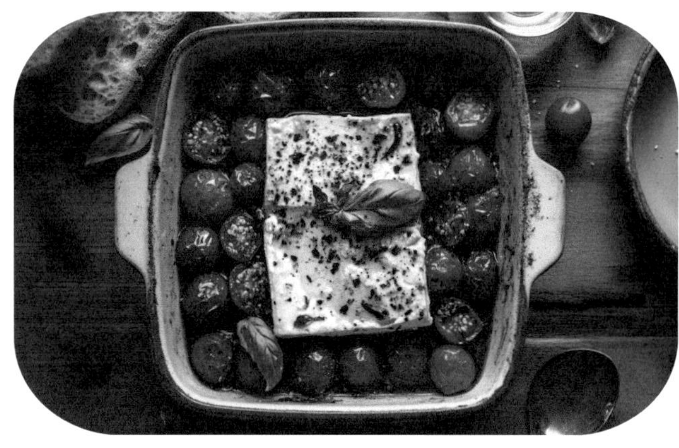

Baked Feta and Cherry Tomatoes

PREPARATION TIME: 5 MINUTES

COOKING TIME: 25 MINUTES

SERVES: 4

Nutrition Information (Per Serving):
210 Calories / 14g Fat / 10g Carbohydrates / 7g Protein / 320mg Sodium / 4g Sugar

INGREDIENTS:

- 1 block (8 oz) feta cheese
- 2 cups cherry tomatoes
- 3 tablespoons olive oil
- 2 garlic cloves, minced
- 1 teaspoon dried oregano
- 1/2 teaspoon red chili flakes (optional)
- Fresh basil leaves for garnish
- Salt and pepper to taste

DIRECTIONS:

1. Preheat the oven to 400°F (200°C).
2. Place the feta block in the center of a small baking dish. Arrange the cherry tomatoes around it.
3. Drizzle olive oil over the feta and tomatoes. Sprinkle with minced garlic, oregano, chili flakes (if using), salt, and pepper.
4. Bake for 20-25 minutes, or until the tomatoes are blistered and the feta is soft and golden on top.
5. Garnish with fresh basil leaves and serve warm as a dip, spread, or topping for crusty bread or pasta.

TIP: Add a squeeze of fresh lemon juice after baking for a zesty flavor boost.

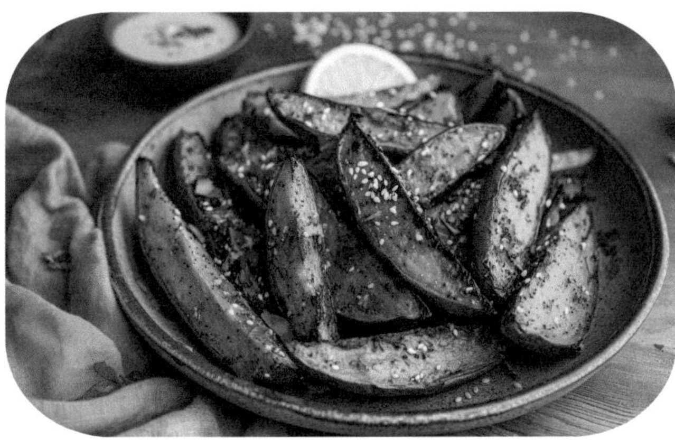

Sweet Potato Wedges with Tahini Sauce

PREPARATION TIME: 5 MINUTES

COOKING TIME: 20-25 MINUTES

SERVES: 4

Nutrition Information (Per Serving):
240 Calories / 12g Fat / 30g Carbohydrates / 4g Protein / 320mg Sodium / 5g Sugar

INGREDIENTS:

- 2-3 large sweet potatoes, cut into wedges
- 2 tablespoons olive oil
- 1 teaspoon smoked paprika
- 1/2 teaspoon ground cumin
- Salt and pepper to taste
- Tahini sauce (see recipe on p. 20)

DIRECTIONS:

1. Preheat the oven to 425°F (220°C) and line a baking sheet with parchment paper.
2. Toss the sweet potato wedges with olive oil, smoked paprika, cumin, salt, and pepper in a large bowl until evenly coated.
3. Spread the wedges on the baking sheet in a single layer. Bake for 20-25 minutes, flipping halfway through, until golden brown and slightly crispy.
4. Arrange the roasted sweet potatoes on a plate, drizzle with tahini sauce, and serve immediately.

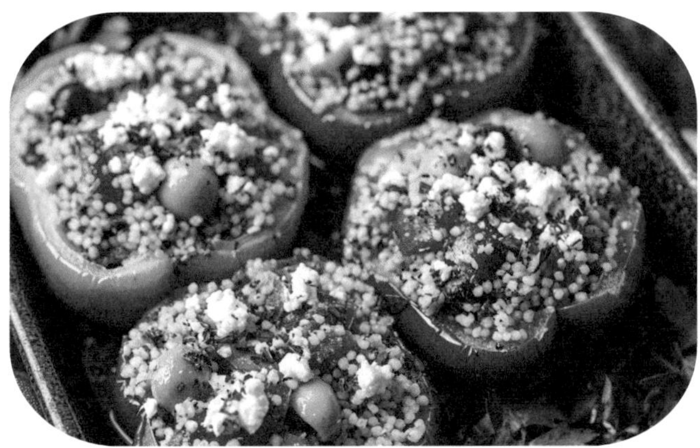

Stuffed Bell Peppers with Couscous

PREPARATION TIME: 10 MINUTES

COOKING TIME: 20 MINUTES

SERVES: 4

Nutrition Information (Per Serving):
240 Calories / 8g Fat / 35g Carbohydrates / 6g Protein / 310mg Sodium / 3g Sugar

INGREDIENTS:

For the Peppers:

- 4 medium bell peppers, halved and seeds removed
- 1 tablespoon olive oil

For the Filling:

- 1 cup couscous
- 1 1/4 cups vegetable broth (or water)
- 1 small onion, finely chopped
- 2 garlic cloves, minced
- 1 medium tomato, diced
- 1/4 cup Kalamata olives, chopped
- 2 tablespoons fresh parsley, chopped
- 1 teaspoon dried oregano
- Salt and pepper to taste
- Crumbled feta cheese (optional)

DIRECTIONS:

1. Preheat the oven to 400°F (200°C). Lightly brush the halved bell peppers with olive oil and place them cut-side up in a baking dish.
2. Bring vegetable broth to a boil in a small pot. Remove from heat, stir in couscous, cover, and let sit for 5 minutes. Fluff with a fork.
3. While the couscous cooks, heat a skillet over medium heat. Sauté the onion and garlic for 2-3 minutes until softened.
4. Combine the cooked couscous with the sautéed onion and garlic, diced tomato, olives, parsley, oregano, salt, and pepper. Mix well.
5. Spoon the couscous mixture evenly into the bell pepper halves.
6. Bake for 15-20 minutes, or until the peppers are tender.
7. Optional: Sprinkle with crumbled feta cheese before serving.

Chapter 5

FISH and SEAFOOD

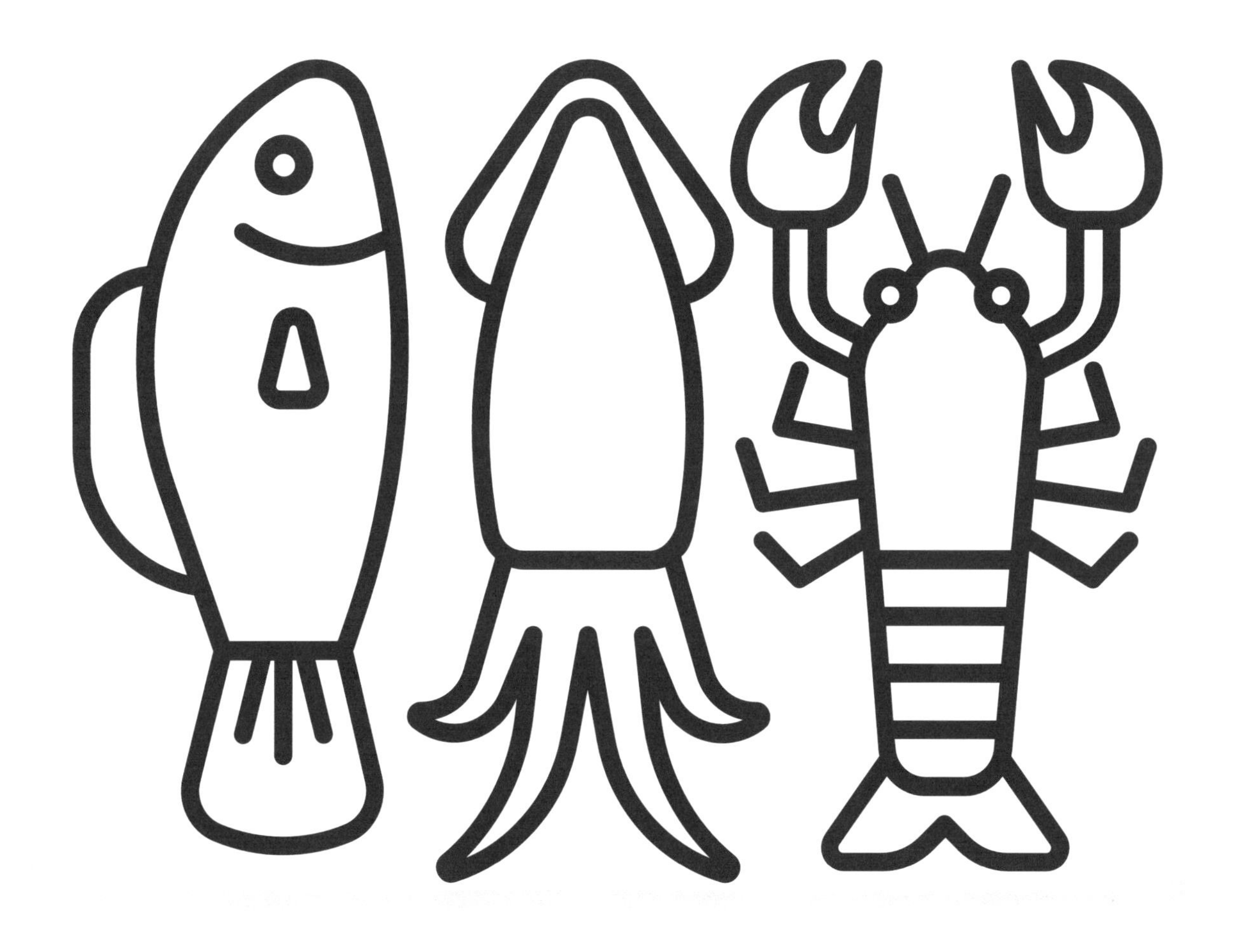

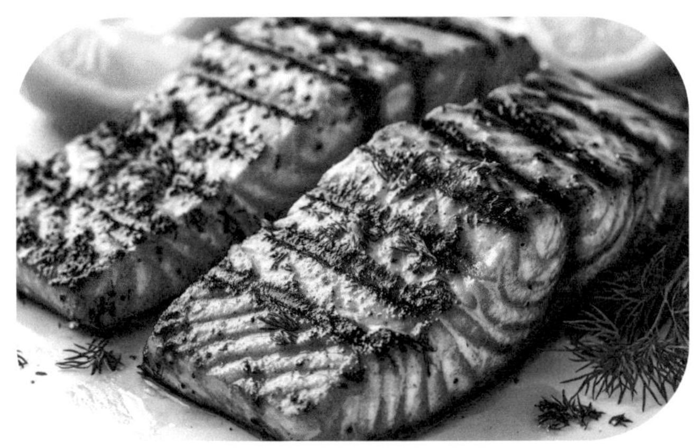

Grilled Salmon with Dill

PREPARATION TIME: 5 MINUTES

MARINATING TIME: 15 MINUTES

COOKING TIME: 10-12 MINUTES

SERVES: 4

Nutrition Information (Per Serving):
320 Calories / 18g Fat / 2g Carbohydrates / 34g Protein / 90mg Sodium / 1g Sugar

INGREDIENTS:

- 4 salmon fillets (about 6 oz each)
- 2 tablespoons olive oil
- Juice of 1 lemon
- 2 tablespoons fresh dill, chopped (or 1 tablespoon dried dill)
- 2 cloves garlic, minced
- Salt and pepper to taste
- Lemon wedges, for serving
- Fresh dill sprigs, for garnish (optional)

DIRECTIONS:

1. Mix olive oil, lemon juice, dill, garlic, salt, and pepper in a bowl.
2. Marinate salmon fillets in the mixture for 15 minutes.
3. Preheat the grill to medium-high heat (375°F to 400°F).
4. Oil the grill grates, then grill the salmon skin-side down for 4-6 minutes per side, until cooked through.
5. Serve with lemon wedges and garnish with fresh dill.

TIP: Serve the salmon with a side of grilled vegetables or a light salad for a complete Mediterranean meal.

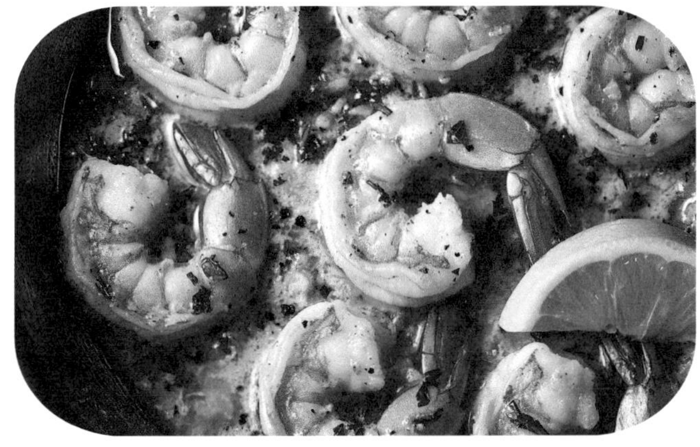

Simple Shrimp Scampi

PREPARATION TIME: 10 MINUTES

COOKING TIME: 10 MINUTES

SERVES: 4

Nutrition Information (Per Serving):
310 Calories / 18g Fat / 7g Carbohydrates / 24g Protein / 400mg Sodium / 1g Sugar

INGREDIENTS:

- 1 lb large shrimp, peeled and deveined
- 3 tablespoons olive oil
- 4 cloves garlic, minced
- 1/4 teaspoon red pepper flakes (optional)
- 1/2 cup dry white wine (or chicken broth)
- Juice of 1 lemon
- 3 tablespoons unsalted butter
- Salt and pepper to taste
- 2 tablespoons fresh parsley, chopped
- 8 oz linguine or spaghetti (optional)
- Lemon wedges, for serving

DIRECTIONS:

1. Cook the pasta according to package instructions if using. Drain and set aside.
2. Heat olive oil in a large skillet over medium-high heat. Add shrimp and cook for 1-2 minutes per side, until pink and opaque. Remove shrimp and set aside.
3. In the same skillet, add garlic and red pepper flakes. Sauté for 30 seconds until fragrant. Add white wine and lemon juice, simmer for 2-3 minutes.
4. Stir in butter until melted. Return shrimp to the skillet and toss to coat in the sauce. Season with salt and pepper.
5. Serve immediately, garnished with fresh parsley and lemon wedges. Toss with pasta if desired.

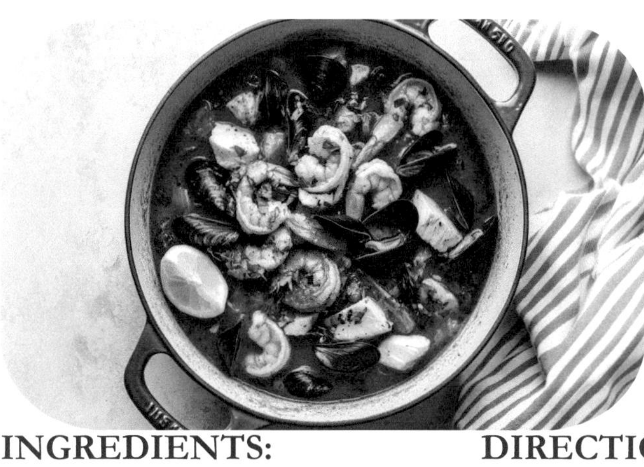

Cioppino (Seafood Stew)

PREPARATION TIME: 5 MINUTES

COOKING TIME: 20 MINUTES

SERVES: 4

Nutrition Information (Per Serving):
320 Calories / 18g Fat / 2g Carbohydrates / 34g Protein / 90mg Sodium / 1g Sugar

INGREDIENTS:

- 2 tablespoons olive oil
- 1 small onion (chopped), 2 garlic cloves (minced), 1 red bell pepper (diced)
- 1 can (14 oz) diced tomatoes, 2 cups fish or vegetable stock
- 1/2 teaspoon smoked paprika, 1/2 teaspoon dried oregano
- 1/2 pound mixed seafood (mussels, shrimp, clams), cleaned
- 1/2 pound white fish fillets (e.g., cod or halibut), cut into chunks
- 2 tablespoons fresh parsley (chopped), juice of 1/2 lemon
- Salt and pepper to taste

DIRECTIONS:

1. Heat olive oil in a large pot over medium heat. Sauté the onion, garlic, and red bell pepper for 3-4 minutes until softened.
2. Stir in the diced tomatoes, broth, smoked paprika, and dried oregano. Bring to a gentle boil and simmer for 5 minutes.
3. Add the white fish chunks and mixed seafood to the pot. Cover and cook for 7-10 minutes until the seafood is cooked through, the shrimp are pink, and the mussels and clams open (discard unopened ones).
4. Stir in the lemon juice, season with salt and pepper, and sprinkle with fresh parsley.
5. Serve warm with crusty bread or over rice.

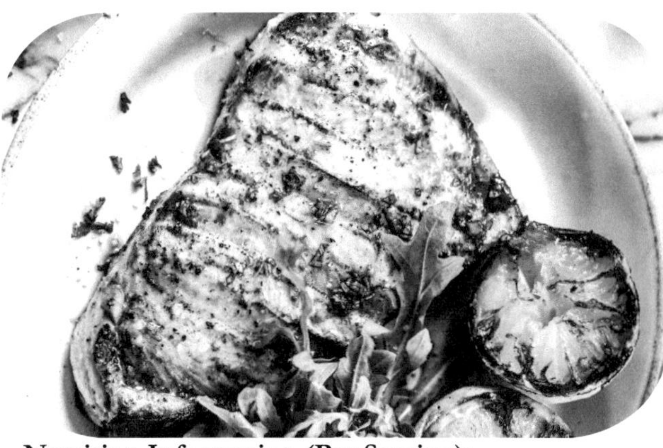

Grilled Mediterranean Swordfish

PREPARATION TIME: 5 MINUTES

MARINATING TIME: 15 MINUTES

COOKING TIME: 10-12 MINUTES

SERVES: 4

Nutrition Information (Per Serving):
320 Calories / 14g Fat / 1g Carbohydrates / 44g Protein / 220mg Sodium / 0g Sugar

INGREDIENTS:

- 4 swordfish steaks (about 1 inch thick)
- 3 tablespoons olive oil
- Juice of 1 lemon
- 2 teaspoons dried oregano
- 2 garlic cloves, minced
- 1 teaspoon paprika
- 1/4 teaspoon chili flakes (optional)
- Salt and pepper to taste
- Fresh parsley and lemon wedges for garnish

DIRECTIONS:

1. Whisk olive oil, lemon juice, oregano, garlic, paprika, chili flakes (if using), salt, and pepper in a small bowl.
2. Marinate swordfish in the mixture for 15 minutes at room temperature.
3. Preheat a grill or grill pan over medium-high heat and lightly oil the grates.
4. Grill swordfish for 4-5 minutes per side until cooked through and grill marks appear.
5. Serve with fresh parsley and lemon wedges. Pair well with grilled vegetables or a fresh salad for a complete meal.

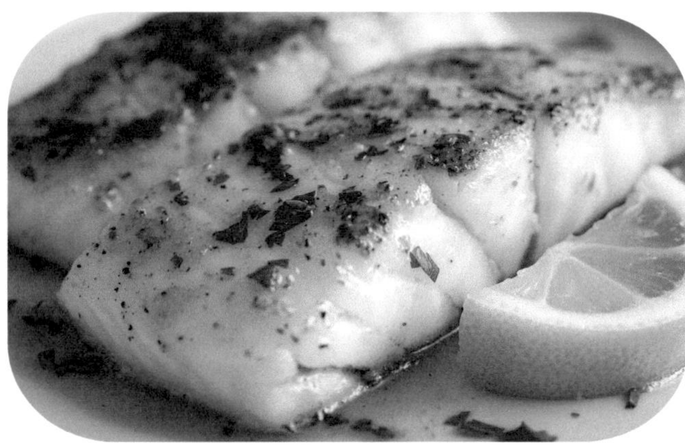

Baked Cod with Lemon

 **PREPARATION TIME:** 5 MINUTES

 **COOKING TIME:** 15-20 MINUTES

 **SERVES:** 4

Nutrition Information (Per Serving):
220 Calories / 9g Fat / 2g Carbohydrates / 32g Protein / 180mg Sodium / 1g Sugar

INGREDIENTS:

- 4 cod fillets (about 6 oz each)
- 2 tablespoons olive oil
- Juice of 1 lemon
- Zest of 1 lemon
- 2 cloves garlic, minced
- 1 teaspoon dried oregano
- Salt and pepper to taste
- Fresh parsley, chopped (optional, for garnish)
- Lemon wedges, for serving

DIRECTIONS:

1. Preheat the oven to 400°F (200°C). Line a baking sheet with parchment paper or lightly grease it.
2. In a small bowl, mix together olive oil, lemon juice, lemon zest, garlic, oregano, salt, and pepper.
3. Place the cod fillets on the prepared baking sheet. Brush the lemon mixture over the fillets, ensuring they are evenly coated.
4. Bake in the preheated oven for 15-20 minutes, or until the cod is opaque and flakes easily with a fork.
5. Serve immediately, garnished with fresh parsley and lemon wedges.

TIP: Pair the baked cod with a Greek salad, roasted vegetables, or herb-roasted potatoes.

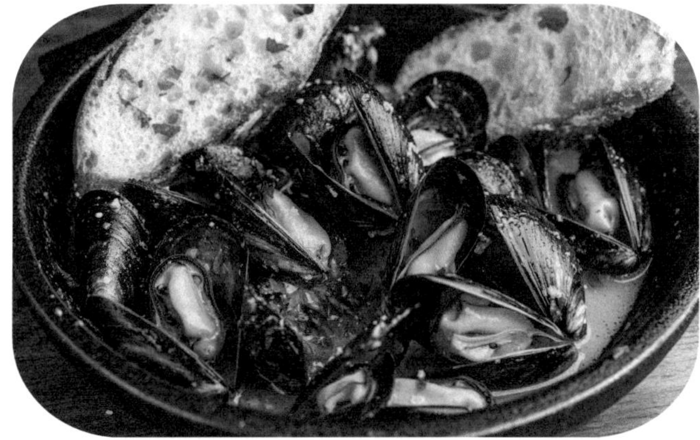

Mussels in White Wine Sauce

 **PREPARATION TIME:** 10 MINUTES

 **COOKING TIME:** 10 MINUTES

 **SERVES:** 4

Nutrition Information (Per Serving):
250 Calories / 10g Fat / 6g Carbohydrates / 30g Protein / 500mg Sodium / 1g Sugar

INGREDIENTS:

- 2 lbs fresh mussels, scrubbed and with beards removed
- 2 tablespoons olive oil
- 4 cloves garlic, minced
- 1 small shallot, finely chopped
- 1 cup dry white wine
- 1/2 cup vegetable or fish broth
- Juice of 1 lemon
- 2 tablespoons unsalted butter
- Salt and pepper to taste
- Fresh parsley, chopped (optional, for garnish)
- Crusty bread, for serving

DIRECTIONS:

1. Heat olive oil in a large, deep skillet or pot over medium heat. Add the minced garlic and chopped shallot, sautéing for 2-3 minutes until softened and fragrant.
2. Pour in the white wine and broth, bringing the mixture to a simmer. Cook for 2 minutes to allow the flavors to meld.
3. Add the cleaned mussels to the skillet, cover, and cook for 5-7 minutes, shaking the pan occasionally, until the mussels have opened. Discard any mussels that do not open.
4. Stir in the lemon juice and butter, allowing the butter to melt into the sauce. Season with salt and pepper to taste.
5. Serve immediately, garnished with fresh parsley and accompanied by crusty bread to soak up the delicious sauce.

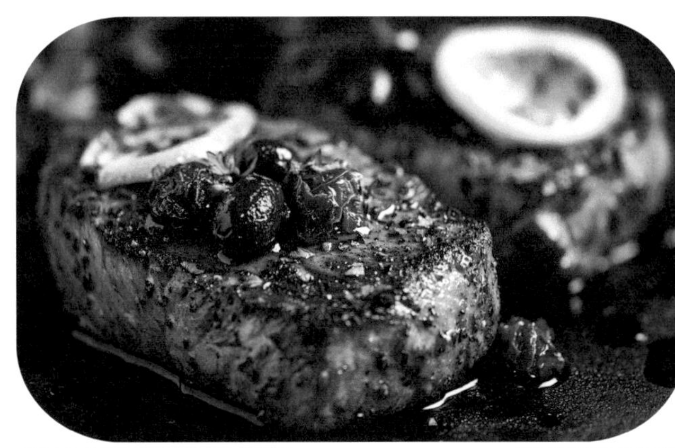

Mediterranean Tuna Steaks

PREPARATION TIME: 5 MINUTES

MARINATING TIME: 15 MINUTES

COOKING TIME: 6-8 MINUTES

SERVES: 4

Nutrition Information (Per Serving):
300 Calories / 15g Fat / 2g Carbohydrates / 38g Protein / 350mg Sodium / 1g Sugar

INGREDIENTS:

- 4 tuna steaks (about 6 oz each)
- 2 tablespoons olive oil
- 2 cloves garlic, minced
- 1 teaspoon dried oregano
- 1 teaspoon dried thyme
- Juice and zest of 1 lemon
- 1/4 cup Kalamata olives, pitted and halved
- 1/4 cup sun-dried tomatoes, chopped
- Salt and pepper to taste
- Fresh parsley, chopped (for garnish)
- Lemon wedges (for serving)

DIRECTIONS:

1. In a small bowl, combine the olive oil, minced garlic, dried oregano, dried thyme, lemon juice, and lemon zest. Mix well. Pat the tuna steaks dry with a paper towel and season both sides with salt and pepper. Brush the lemon-herb mixture over both sides of the tuna steaks, ensuring they are evenly coated. Let the tuna steaks marinate for 15 minutes.
2. Heat a large skillet or grill pan over medium-high heat. Once hot, add the tuna steaks and cook for 2-3 minutes per side, or until they reach your desired level of doneness (tuna is best served slightly pink in the center).
3. In the last minute of cooking, add the Kalamata olives and sun-dried tomatoes to the pan to warm them slightly.
4. Remove the tuna steaks from the pan and let them rest for a minute before serving.
5. Garnish the tuna steaks with fresh parsley and serve with lemon wedges on the side.

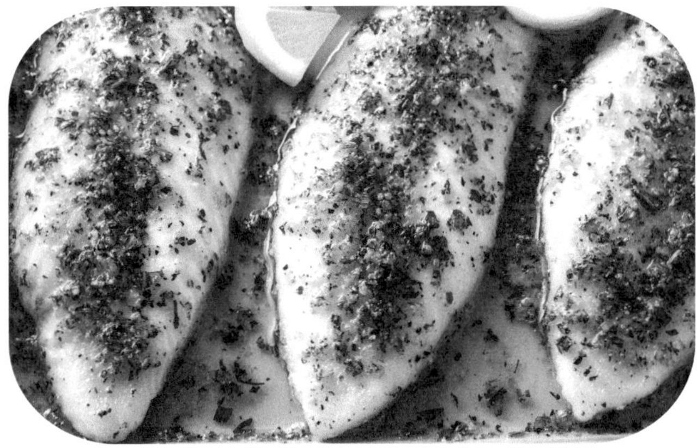

Lemon Herb Tilapia

PREPARATION TIME: 5 MINUTES

MARINATING TIME: 10-15MINUTES (optional but recommended)

COOKING TIME: 10 -12 MINUTES

SERVES: 4

Nutrition Information (Per Serving):
230 Calories / 11g Fat / 2g Carbohydrates / 30g Protein / 240mg Sodium / 0g Sugar

INGREDIENTS:

- 4 tilapia fillets (about 6 oz each)
- 2 tablespoons olive oil
- Juice and zest of 1 lemon
- 2 cloves garlic, minced
- 1 teaspoon dried thyme
- 1 teaspoon dried oregano
- Salt and pepper to taste
- Fresh parsley, chopped (optional, for garnish)
- Lemon wedges, for serving

DIRECTIONS:

1. Preheat the oven to 400°F (200°C). Lightly grease a baking dish or line it with parchment paper.
2. In a small bowl, mix together the olive oil, lemon juice, lemon zest, garlic, thyme, oregano, salt, and pepper.
3. Place the tilapia fillets in the prepared baking dish. Brush the lemon herb mixture over the fillets, ensuring they are evenly coated. Allow the fillets to marinate for 10-15 minutes for better flavor.
4. Place the baking dish in the preheated oven and bake for 10-12 minutes, or until the tilapia is opaque and flakes easily with a fork.
5. Remove from the oven and serve immediately. Garnish with fresh parsley and lemon wedges on the side.

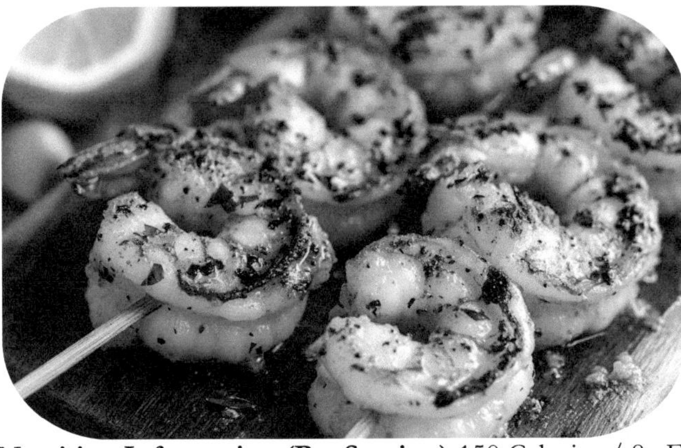

Garlic Lemon Shrimp Skewers

PREPARATION TIME: 5 MINUTES

MARINATING TIME: 15 MINUTES

COOKING TIME: 5-7 MINUTES

SERVES: 4

Nutrition Information (Per Serving):150 Calories / 8g Fat / 3g Carbohydrates / 20g Protein / 220mg Sodium / 1g Sugar

INGREDIENTS:

- 1 pound large shrimp, peeled and deveined
- 2 tablespoons olive oil
- 2 cloves garlic, minced
- 1 lemon, juiced
- 1 tablespoon fresh parsley, chopped
- Salt and pepper, to taste

DIRECTIONS:

1. If using wooden skewers, soak them in water for at least 15 minutes to prevent them from burning on the grill.
2. In a bowl, combine the olive oil, minced garlic, lemon juice, and chopped parsley. Add the shrimp, season with salt and pepper, and toss to coat evenly. Let the shrimp marinate for 15 minutes to absorb the flavors.
3. Thread the marinated shrimp onto the soaked skewers.
4. Preheat a grill or grill pan over medium-high heat. Cook the shrimp skewers for about 2-3 minutes on each side, or until the shrimp are pink and opaque.
5. Remove from the grill and serve immediately with a wedge of lemon on the side.

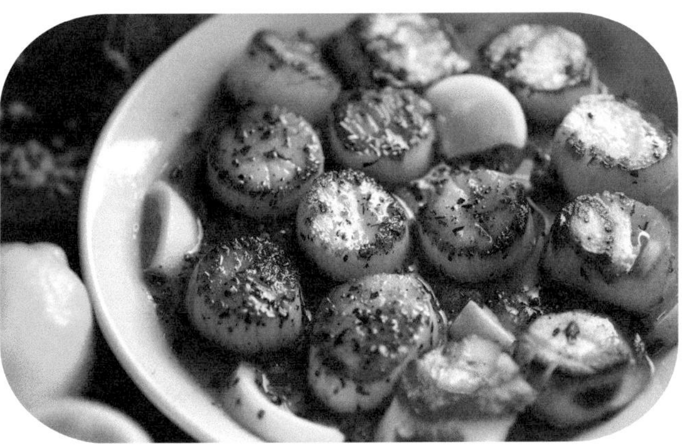

Garlic Butter Scallops

PREPARATION TIME: 10 MINUTES

COOKING TIME: 5-7 MINUTES

SERVES: 4

Nutrition Information (Per Serving):
220 Calories / 15g Fat / 6g Carbohydrates / 18g Protein / 400mg Sodium / 0g Sugar

INGREDIENTS:

- 1 lb large scallops, patted dry
- 3 tablespoons unsalted butter
- 4 cloves garlic, minced
- 2 tablespoons olive oil
- Juice of 1/2 lemon
- Salt and pepper to taste
- Fresh parsley, chopped (optional, for garnish)
- Lemon wedges, for serving

DIRECTIONS:

1. Season the scallops with salt and pepper on both sides.
2. Heat 2 tablespoons of butter and the olive oil in a large skillet over medium-high heat. Add the scallops in a single layer and cook for 2-3 minutes on each side, until golden brown and opaque. Remove the scallops from the skillet and set aside.
3. In the same skillet, add the remaining tablespoon of butter and the minced garlic. Sauté for 1 minute until fragrant.
4. Add the lemon juice and stir to combine. Return the scallops to the skillet, tossing them in the garlic butter sauce to coat.
5. Serve immediately, garnished with fresh parsley and lemon wedges.

TIP: Pair these scallops with a light salad, steamed vegetables, or a side of your choice of pasta.

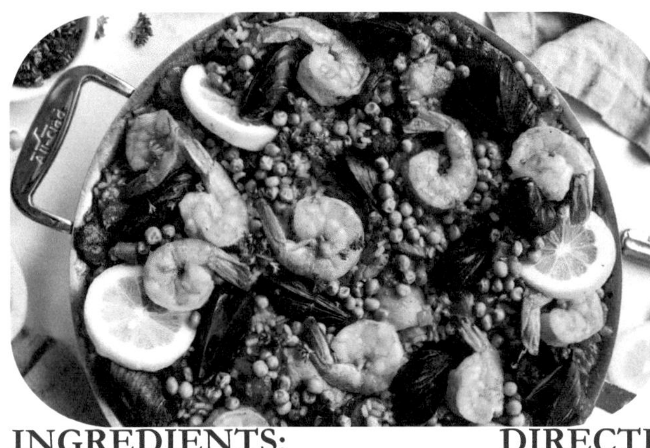

Seafood Paella (Quick Version)

PREPARATION TIME: 10 MINUTES

COOKING TIME: 20 MINUTES

SERVES: 4

Nutrition Information (Per Serving):
350 Calories / 10g Fat / 40g Carbohydrates / 25g Protein / 500mg Sodium / 3g Sugar

INGREDIENTS:

- 2 tbsp olive oil
- 1 small onion (chopped), 2 garlic cloves (minced)
- 1 red bell pepper (diced)
- 1 cup Arborio or short-grain rice
- 2 1/2 cups chicken or seafood stock
- 1/4 tsp saffron threads (optional)
- 1/2 tsp smoked paprika
- 1/2 lb mixed seafood (shrimp, mussels, clams), cleaned
- 1/2 lb white fish (cod or halibut), cut into chunks
- 1/2 cup frozen peas, juice of 1/2 lemon
- 2 tbsp fresh parsley (chopped)
- Salt and pepper to taste

DIRECTIONS:

1. Heat olive oil in a large skillet or paella pan over medium heat. Sauté the onion, garlic, and red bell pepper for 3-4 minutes until softened.
2. Add the rice to the skillet and stir to coat with the oil. Cook for 1-2 minutes.
3. Pour in the stock, saffron (if using), and smoked paprika. Stir well, bring to a boil, then reduce the heat to a simmer. Cover and cook for 10 minutes.
4. Arrange the mixed seafood and white fish chunks on top of the rice. Scatter the peas over the dish. Cover and cook for an additional 8-10 minutes, or until the seafood is cooked through and the rice is tender.
5. Remove from heat, drizzle with lemon juice, and garnish with fresh parsley. Season with salt and pepper to taste.
6. Serve warm directly from the skillet for an authentic presentation.

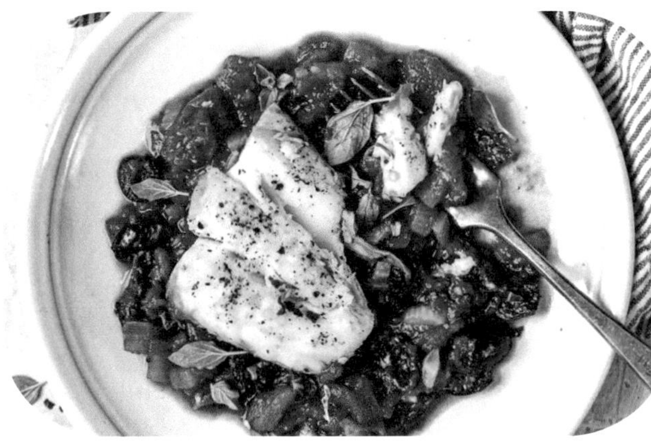

Baked Sea Bass with Tomatoes

PREPARATION TIME: 5 MINUTES

COOKING TIME: 25-30 MINUTES

SERVES: 4

Nutrition Information (Per Serving):
280 Calories / 12g Fat / 4g Carbohydrates / 36g Protein / 350mg Sodium / 3g Sugar

INGREDIENTS:

- 4 sea bass fillets (about 6 oz each)
- 2 tablespoons olive oil
- 2 cups cherry tomatoes, halved
- 2 cloves garlic, minced
- 1/4 cup Kalamata olives, pitted and halved (optional)
- 1/4 cup dry white wine (optional)
- 1 teaspoon dried oregano
- 1 teaspoon dried thyme
- Juice of 1 lemon
- Salt and pepper to taste
- Fresh basil or parsley, chopped (optional, for garnish)
- Lemon wedges, for serving

DIRECTIONS:

1. Preheat your oven to 400°F (200°C). Lightly grease a baking dish with olive oil.
2. Place the sea bass fillets in the baking dish. Season with salt, pepper, and lemon juice.
3. In a small bowl, mix together the cherry tomatoes, garlic, olives, white wine (if using), oregano, and thyme. Spoon this mixture over and around the sea bass fillets.
4. Bake in the preheated oven for 25-30 minutes, or until the sea bass is opaque and flakes easily with a fork.
5. Serve the sea bass topped with the baked tomatoes and garnished with fresh basil or parsley. Serve with lemon wedges on the side.

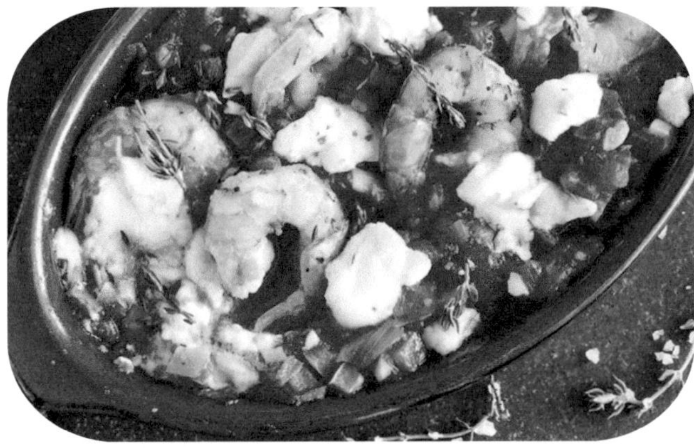

Baked Shrimp with Tomatos and Feta

PREPARATION TIME: 10 MINUTES

COOKING TIME: 15-20 MINUTES

SERVES: 4

Nutrition Information (Per Serving):
290 Calories / 15g Fat / 6g Carbohydrates / 30g Protein / 480mg Sodium / 3g Sugar

INGREDIENTS:

- 1 lb large shrimp, peeled and deveined
- 2 tablespoons olive oil
- 3 cloves garlic, minced
- 1 can (14.5 oz) diced tomatoes
- 1/4 cup dry white wine (optional)
- 1 teaspoon dried oregano
- 1/2 teaspoon red pepper flakes (optional)
- Salt and pepper to taste
- 1/2 cup crumbled feta cheese
- 2 tablespoons fresh parsley, chopped (optional, for garnish)
- Lemon wedges, for serving

DIRECTIONS:

1. Preheat your oven to 375°F (190°C). Lightly grease a baking dish with olive oil.
2. In a skillet, heat the olive oil over medium heat. Add the minced garlic and sauté for 1 minute until fragrant.
3. Add the diced tomatoes (with their juice), white wine (if using), oregano, red pepper flakes (if using), salt, and pepper. Simmer for 5 minutes, allowing the flavors to meld.
4. Arrange the shrimp in the baking dish. Pour the tomato mixture over the shrimp, then sprinkle the crumbled feta cheese on top.
5. Bake in the preheated oven for 15-20 minutes, or until the shrimp are pink and opaque, and the feta is slightly melted.
6. Serve immediately, garnished with fresh parsley and lemon wedges.

Calamari with Lemon and Garlic

PREPARATION TIME: 10 MINUTES

COOKING TIME: 5 MINUTES

SERVES: 4

Nutrition Information (Per Serving):
200 Calories / 10g Fat / 4g Carbohydrates / 22g Protein / 380mg Sodium / 1g Sugar

INGREDIENTS:

- 1 lb calamari, cleaned and cut into rings
- 3 tablespoons olive oil
- 3 cloves garlic, minced
- Juice of 1 lemon
- 1 teaspoon dried oregano
- Salt and pepper to taste
- Fresh parsley, chopped (optional, for garnish)
- Lemon wedges, for serving

DIRECTIONS:

1. Heat the olive oil in a large skillet over medium-high heat. Add the minced garlic and sauté for 1 minute until fragrant.
2. Add the calamari rings to the skillet. Cook for 2-3 minutes, stirring frequently, until the calamari is opaque and tender.
3. Stir in the lemon juice, oregano, salt, and pepper. Cook for an additional 1-2 minutes to combine the flavors.
4. Serve immediately, garnished with fresh parsley and lemon wedges on the side.

TIP: Serve this dish with a side of fresh salad, grilled vegetables, or a light pasta.

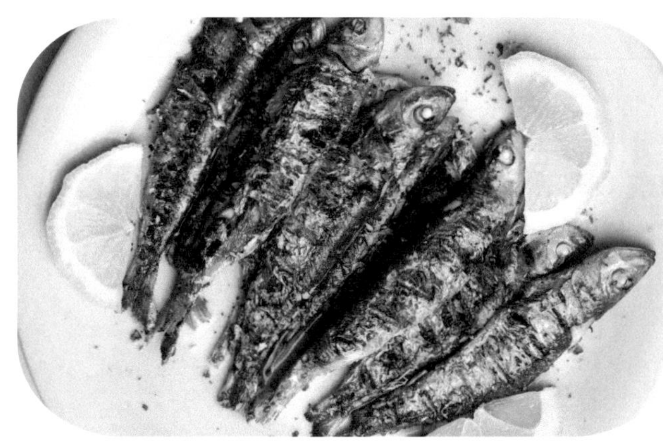

Sardines with Lemon and Herbs

PREPARATION TIME: 10 MINUTES

COOKING TIME: 10 MINUTES

SERVES: 4

Nutrition Information (Per Serving):
180 Calories / 10g Fat / 2g Carbohydrates / 20g Protein / 250mg Sodium / 1g Sugar

INGREDIENTS:

- 1 lb fresh sardines, cleaned and gutted
- 2 tablespoons olive oil
- Juice and zest of 1 lemon
- 2 cloves garlic, minced
- 1 teaspoon dried oregano
- 1 teaspoon dried thyme
- Salt and pepper to taste
- Fresh parsley, chopped (for garnish)
- Lemon wedges, for serving

DIRECTIONS:

1. Preheat your grill or broiler to medium-high heat.
2. In a small bowl, mix olive oil, lemon juice, lemon zest, garlic, oregano, thyme, salt, and pepper.
3. Brush the sardines with the lemon herb mixture on both sides.
4. Grill or broil the sardines for 3-4 minutes on each side, until they are cooked through and slightly charred.
5. Serve immediately, garnished with fresh parsley and lemon wedges.

TIP: Serve these sardines with a side of grilled vegetables or a light salad.

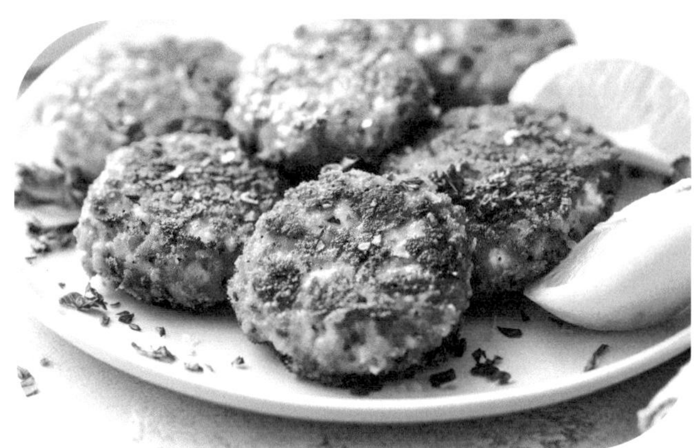

Salmon Patties

PREPARATION TIME: 10 MINUTES

COOKING TIME: 15 MINUTES

SERVES: 4

Nutrition Information (Per Serving):
250 Calories / 14g Fat / 8g Carbohydrates / 22g Protein / 350mg Sodium / 1g Sugar

INGREDIENTS:

- 1 can (14.75 oz) salmon, drained and flaked
- 1/2 cup breadcrumbs
- 1/4 cup finely chopped onion
- 1 egg, beaten
- 2 tablespoons fresh parsley, chopped
- 1 tablespoon mayonnaise
- 1 tablespoon Dijon mustard
- 1/2 teaspoon garlic powder
- Salt and pepper to taste
- 2 tablespoons olive oil (for frying)
- Lemon wedges, for serving

DIRECTIONS:

1. In a large bowl, combine the salmon, breadcrumbs, onion, egg, parsley, mayonnaise, Dijon mustard, garlic powder, salt, and pepper. Mix until well combined.
2. Form the mixture into 4 patties.
3. Heat the olive oil in a skillet over medium heat. Cook the patties for 3-4 minutes on each side, or until golden brown and cooked through.
4. Serve hot with lemon wedges.

TIP: These salmon patties are also delicious in a sandwich with fresh greens and a dollop of Tzatziki Dip.

Chapter 6

MEAT and POULTRY

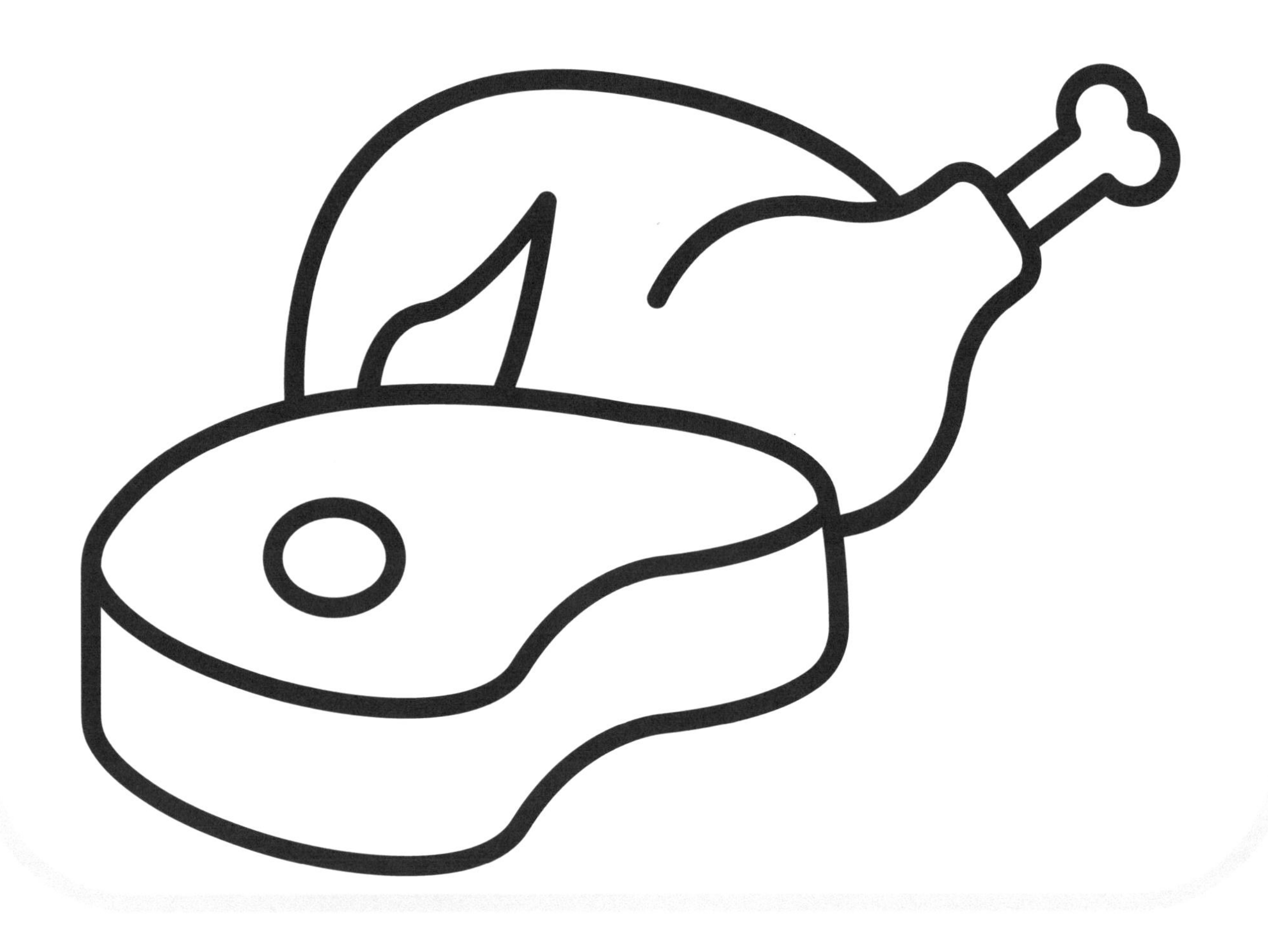

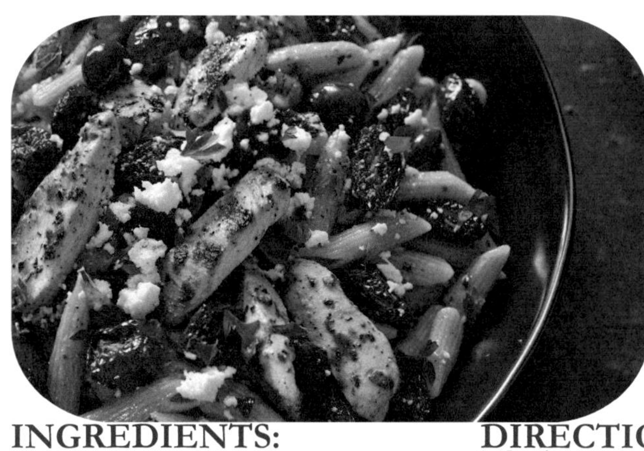

Mediterranean Chicken Pasta

PREPARATION TIME: 10 MINUTES

COOKING TIME: 20 MINUTES

SERVES: 4

Nutrition Information (Per Serving):
410 Calories / 15g Fat / 38g Carbohydrates / 30g Protein / 520mg Sodium / 4g Sugar

INGREDIENTS:

- 2 tablespoons olive oil
- 2 chicken breasts, sliced into strips
- 3 garlic cloves, minced
- 1/2 teaspoon dried oregano
- 1/2 teaspoon smoked paprika
- 12 oz penne or your choice of pasta
- 1 cup cherry tomatoes, halved
- 1/3 cup Kalamata olives, sliced
- 1/4 cup sun-dried tomatoes, chopped
- 1/3 cup crumbled feta cheese
- 2 tablespoons fresh parsley, chopped
- Juice of 1/2 lemon
- Salt and pepper to taste

DIRECTIONS:

1. Cook pasta according to package instructions. Drain and set aside, reserving 1/2 cup of pasta water.
2. Heat olive oil in a large skillet over medium heat. Season the chicken strips with salt, pepper, oregano, and smoked paprika. Sear the chicken for 4-5 minutes per side, until golden and fully cooked. Remove and set aside.
3. In the same skillet, add minced garlic and sauté for 1 minute until fragrant. Add cherry tomatoes, Kalamata olives, and sun-dried tomatoes. Cook for 3-4 minutes until the tomatoes soften slightly.
4. Return the cooked chicken to the skillet. Stir in the cooked pasta and reserved pasta water to create a light sauce. Toss until evenly combined.
5. Remove from heat and mix in crumbled feta cheese, fresh parsley, and a squeeze of lemon juice. Adjust seasoning with salt and pepper if needed.
6. Serve immediately, garnished with extra parsley or feta if desired.

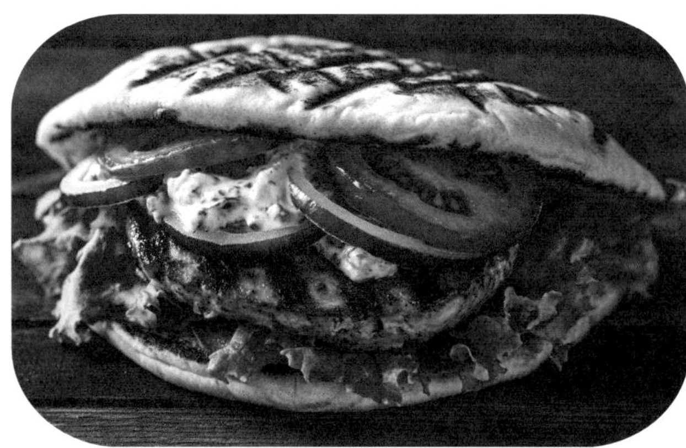

Herbed Burgers with Tzatziki

PREPARATION 10 MINUTES

COOKING TIME: 20-25 MINUTES

SERVES: 4

Nutrition Information (Per Serving):
320 Calories / 15g Fat / 2g Carbohydrates / 40g Protein / 350mg Sodium / 1g Sugar

INGREDIENTS:

- 1 lb ground turkey or beef
- 1/3 cup breadcrumbs
- 1 egg
- 2 tablespoons fresh parsley, chopped
- 2 garlic cloves, minced
- 1 teaspoon dried oregano
- 1/2 teaspoon ground cumin
- Salt and pepper to taste
- 1 tablespoon olive oil (for cooking)
- 1 cup Tzatziki Sauce (see recipe on p.19)
- 4 burger buns or pita bread
- Lettuce, tomato slices, and red onion rings (optional)

DIRECTIONS:

1. In a large bowl, combine the ground turkey or beef, breadcrumbs, egg, parsley, garlic, oregano, cumin, salt, and pepper. Mix until well combined. Shape the mixture into 4 patties.
2. Heat olive oil in a skillet or grill pan over medium heat. Add the patties and cook for 5-6 minutes per side, or until fully cooked (internal temperature of 165°F for turkey, 160°F for beef).
3. Toast the burger buns or pita bread. Spread tzatziki sauce on the bottom bun or pita bread add lettuce, tomato slices, and red onion rings, and top with the cooked patty. Add more tzatziki sauce and cover with the top bun or bread.
4. Serve warm with a side of salad, or grilled vegetables.

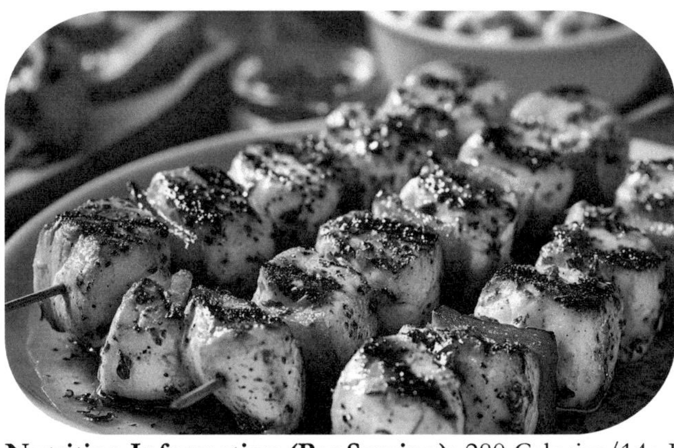

Mediterranean Chicken Skewers

PREPARATION TIME: 5 MINUTES

MARINATING TIME: 10 MINUTES

COOKING TIME: 10 - 15 MINUTES

SERVES: 4

Nutrition Information (Per Serving): 280 Calories/14g Fat/8g Carbohydrates/30g Protein /320mg Sodium/1g Sugar

INGREDIENTS:

- 1 lb chicken breast, cut into 1-inch cubes
- 2 tablespoons olive oil
- Juice of 1 lemon
- 1 tablespoon dried oregano
- 1 red bell pepper, cut into 1-inch pieces
- Salt and pepper, to taste

DIRECTIONS:

1. In a bowl, mix the chicken cubes with olive oil, lemon juice, oregano, salt, and pepper. Cover and let the chicken marinate for 10 minutes while you prepare the grill or skewers.
2. Thread the marinated chicken and bell pepper pieces alternately onto skewers.
3. Preheat a grill or grill pan over medium-high heat. Cook the skewers for 10-12 minutes, turning occasionally, until the chicken is fully cooked and has nice grill marks.
4. Serve hot, garnished with a squeeze of fresh lemon juice, if desired. Pair with a side of tzatziki or a fresh Greek salad for a complete Mediterranean meal.

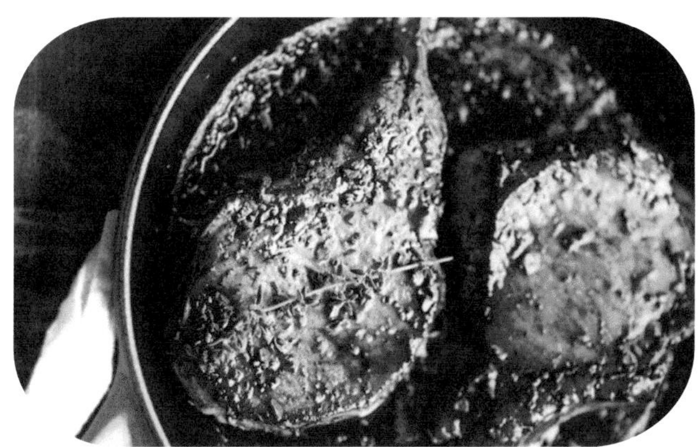

Italian Balsamic Glazed Pork Chops

PREPARATION TIME: 10 MINUTES

COOKING TIME: 15-20 MINUTES

SERVES: 4

Nutrition Information (Per Serving):
330 Calories / 18g Fat / 10g Carbohydrates / 32g Protein / 280mg Sodium / 8g Sugar

INGREDIENTS:

- 4 bone-in pork chops (about 1-inch thick)
- 2 tablespoons olive oil
- 3 garlic cloves, minced
- 1/4 cup balsamic vinegar
- 2 tablespoons honey or maple syrup
- 1 tablespoon Dijon mustard
- 1/4 teaspoon dried thyme
- Salt and pepper, to taste
- Fresh parsley or thyme, chopped (optional, for garnish)

DIRECTIONS:

1. Pat the pork chops dry and season both sides with salt and pepper.
2. Heat olive oil in a large skillet over medium-high heat. Add the pork chops and sear for 3-4 minutes per side, until golden brown. Remove the chops from the skillet and set aside.
3. In the same skillet, lower the heat to medium and add the minced garlic. Sauté for 1 minute until fragrant.
4. Add the balsamic vinegar, honey, Dijon mustard, and thyme to the skillet. Stir to combine, then let the mixture simmer for 2-3 minutes until slightly thickened.
5. Return the pork chops to the skillet and spoon the glaze over the top. Cook for another 5-7 minutes, flipping halfway through, until the pork chops are fully cooked (internal temperature of 145°F/63°C).
6. Serve immediately. Pair with roasted vegetables or a simple arugula salad for a quick and flavorful Mediterranean-inspired meal.

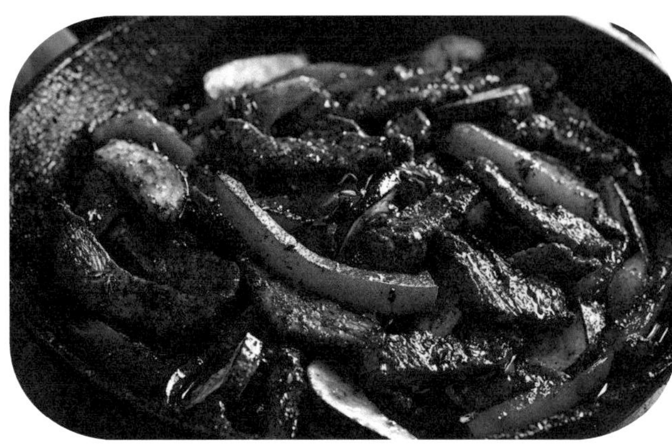

Mediterranean Beef Stir-Fry

PREPARATION TIME: 10 MINUTES

COOKING TIME: 8-10 MINUTES

SERVES: 2

Nutrition Information (Per Serving):
180 Calories / 12g Fat / 8g Carbohydrates / 6g Protein / 220mg Sodium / 3g Sugar

INGREDIENTS:

- 1 lb beef strips (sirloin or flank steak)
- 1 red bell pepper, sliced
- 1 zucchini, sliced
- 2 tablespoons olive oil
- 1 teaspoon dried oregano
- Salt and pepper, to taste

DIRECTIONS:

1. In a large skillet or wok, heat the olive oil over medium-high heat.
2. Add the beef strips to the skillet and stir-fry for about 5-7 minutes, or until browned and cooked through. Remove the beef from the skillet and set aside.
3. In the same skillet, add the sliced red bell pepper and zucchini. Stir-fry for about 5 minutes, or until the vegetables are tender but still crisp.
4. Return the cooked beef to the skillet with the vegetables. Sprinkle with dried oregano and season with salt and pepper to taste. Stir well to combine and cook for an additional 2-3 minutes to heat everything through.

TIP: For added flavor, squeeze a little fresh lemon juice over the stir-fry just before serving. Pair this dish with a side of couscous or quinoa to complete the meal.

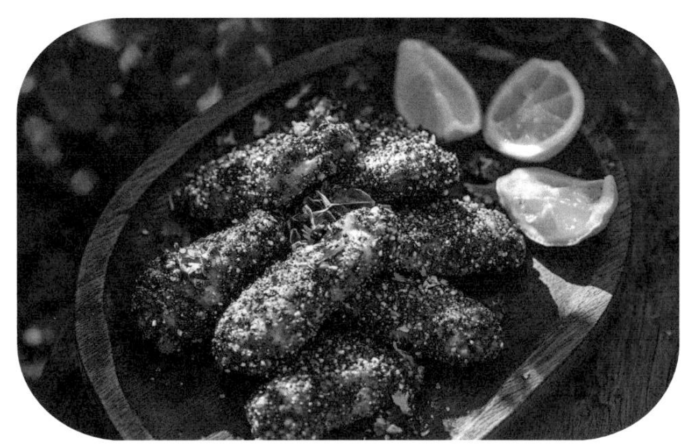

Za'atar Spiced Chicken Wings

PREPARATION TIME: 5 MINUTES

COOKING TIME: 20-25 MINUTES

SERVES: 4

Nutrition Information (Per Serving):
350 Calories / 24g Fat / 2g Carbohydrates / 30g Protein / 400mg Sodium / 1g Sugar

INGREDIENTS:

- 2 lbs chicken wings, trimmed and separated
- 2 tablespoons olive oil
- 2 tablespoons za'atar spice blend
- 1 teaspoon garlic powder
- 1 teaspoon smoked paprika
- Salt and pepper to taste
- 1 lemon, cut into wedges (for serving)

DIRECTIONS:

1. Preheat the oven to 400°F (200°C). Line a baking sheet with parchment paper or foil.
2. In a large bowl, toss the chicken wings with olive oil, za'atar, garlic powder, smoked paprika, salt, and pepper until evenly coated.
3. Spread the wings in a single layer on the prepared baking sheet.
4. Bake for 20-25 minutes, flipping halfway through, until the wings are golden and crispy.
5. Serve warm with lemon wedges for squeezing over the wings.

TIP: Garnish with fresh parsley or lemon zest for an extra burst of flavor.

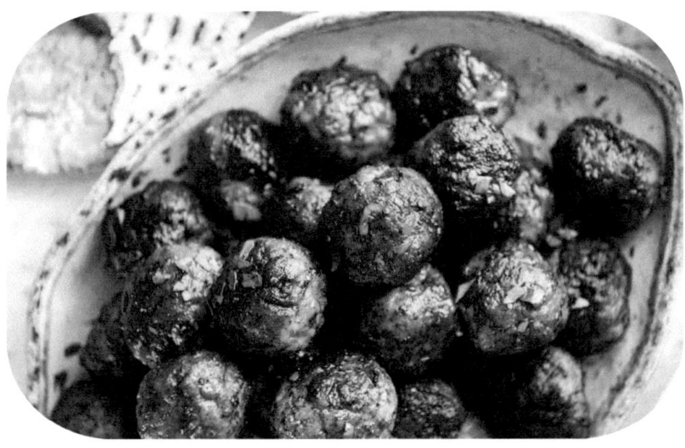

Keftedes (Greek Meatballs)

PREPARATION TIME: 15 MINUTES

COOKING TIME: 20 MINUTES

SERVES: 4-6

Nutrition Information (Per Serving):
250 Calories / 14g Fat / 8g Carbohydrates / 22g Protein / 400mg Sodium / 2g Sugar

INGREDIENTS:

- 1 lb ground beef or a mix of beef and lamb
- 1 small onion, finely chopped
- 2 cloves garlic, minced
- 1/4 cup fresh parsley, chopped
- 1/4 cup fresh mint, chopped (optional)
- 1/4 cup breadcrumbs
- 1 egg, beaten
- 1 teaspoon dried oregano
- 1 teaspoon ground cumin
- Salt and pepper to taste
- 2 tablespoons olive oil (for frying)
- Lemon wedges, for serving

DIRECTIONS:

1. In a large bowl, mix together the ground meat, onion, garlic, parsley, mint (if using), breadcrumbs, egg, oregano, cumin, salt, and pepper until fully combined.
2. Roll the mixture into small meatballs, about 1 to 1.5 inches in diameter.
3. Heat olive oil in a large skillet over medium heat. Cook the meatballs in batches, turning to brown all sides, until they're cooked through, about 8-10 minutes.
4. Once cooked, transfer the meatballs to a paper towel-lined plate to drain excess oil.
5. Serve warm with lemon wedges on the side.

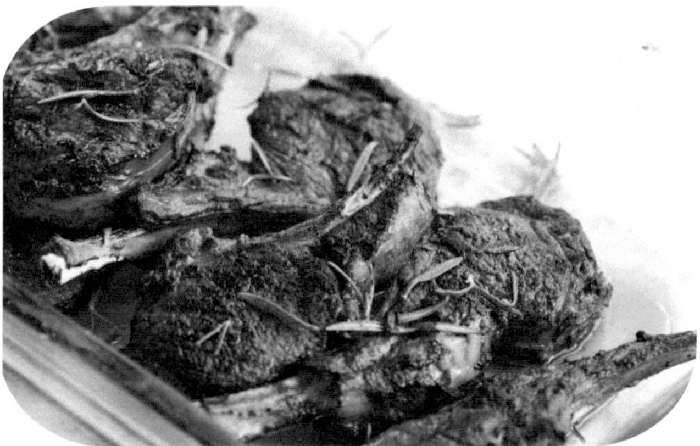

Rosemary Lamb Chops

PREPARATION TIME: 10 MINUTES

COOKING TIME: 15-20 MINUTES

SERVES: 4

Nutrition Information (Per Serving):
320 Calories / 20g Fat / 1g Carbohydrates / 28g Protein / 400mg Sodium / 0g Sugar

INGREDIENTS:

- 8 lamb chops (about 1-inch thick)
- 2 tablespoons olive oil
- 2 cloves garlic, minced
- 2 tablespoons fresh rosemary, chopped (or 1 tablespoon dried rosemary)
- Salt and pepper to taste
- Lemon wedges, for serving

DIRECTIONS:

1. Preheat the oven to 400°F (200°C).
2. In a small bowl, mix the olive oil, garlic, rosemary, salt, and pepper.
3. Rub the rosemary mixture evenly over both sides of the lamb chops.
4. Heat a large ovenproof skillet over medium-high heat. Sear the lamb chops for 2-3 minutes per side until browned.
5. Transfer the skillet to the oven and roast for 8-10 minutes for medium-rare, or longer if desired.
6. Let the lamb chops rest for a few minutes before serving with lemon wedges.

TIP: Pair this dish with a light salad or grilled asparagus with lemon.

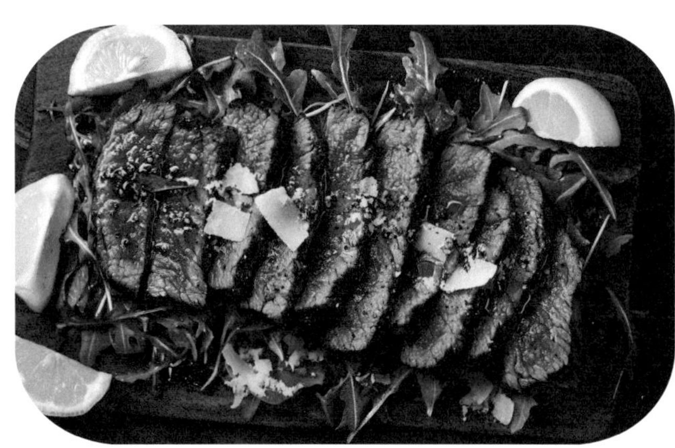

Beef Tagliata (Italian Sliced Steak)

PREPARATION TIME: 10 MINUTES

COOKING TIME: 10-12 MINUTES

SERVES: 4

Nutrition Information (Per Serving):
350 Calories / 22g Fat / 2g Carbohydrates / 32g Protein / 500mg Sodium / 1g Sugar

INGREDIENTS:

- 1.5 lbs ribeye or sirloin steak
- 2 tablespoons olive oil
- Salt and pepper to taste
- 1 tablespoon fresh rosemary, chopped (optional)
- 1 tablespoon fresh thyme, chopped (optional)
- 2 cups arugula
- 1/4 cup shaved Parmesan cheese
- 1 tablespoon balsamic vinegar
- Lemon wedges, for serving

DIRECTIONS:

1. Rub the steak with olive oil, and season generously with salt, pepper, rosemary, and thyme on both sides.
2. Heat a large skillet or grill pan over high heat. Once hot, add the steak and cook for 3-4 minutes per side for medium-rare, or until it reaches your desired doneness. Adjust cooking time for thicker cuts or preferred doneness. Remove the steak from the skillet and let it rest for 5 minutes.
3. While the steak is resting, arrange the arugula on a serving platter. Drizzle with a bit of olive oil and balsamic vinegar.
4. Thinly slice the steak against the grain. Place the slices over the arugula. Top with shaved Parmesan and a squeeze of lemon juice. Serve immediately with lemon wedges on the side.

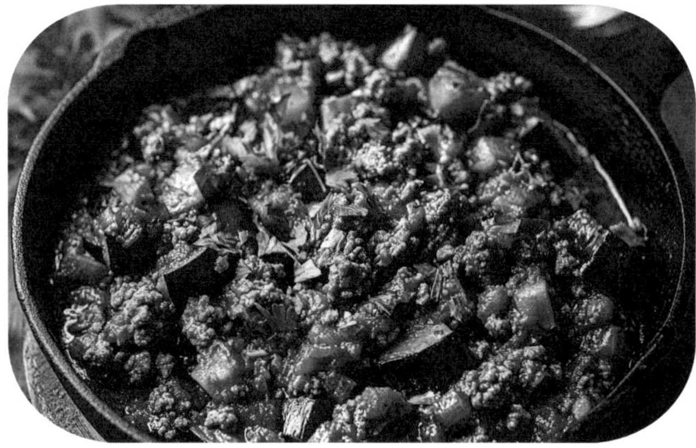

Beef and Eggplant Skillet

PREPARATION TIME: 10 MINUTES

COOKING TIME: 20 MINUTES

SERVES: 4

Nutrition Information (Per Serving):
310 Calories / 18g Fat / 14g Carbohydrates / 23g Protein / 420mg Sodium / 6g Sugar

INGREDIENTS:

- 1 lb ground beef
- 1 medium eggplant, diced
- 1 medium onion, chopped
- 2 garlic cloves, minced
- 1 can (14 oz) diced tomatoes
- 2 tablespoons olive oil
- 1 teaspoon dried oregano
- 1/2 teaspoon smoked paprika
- Salt and pepper, to taste
- Fresh parsley, chopped (optional, for garnish)

DIRECTIONS:

1. Heat olive oil in a large skillet over medium heat. Add the diced eggplant and cook for 5 minutes until softened. Remove and set aside.
2. In the same skillet, cook the ground beef over medium heat, breaking it up with a spoon, until browned. Drain any excess fat if necessary.
3. Add the chopped onion and garlic to the skillet with the beef. Sauté for 2-3 minutes until fragrant.
4. Stir in the diced tomatoes (with their juice), oregano, smoked paprika, salt, and pepper. Return the cooked eggplant to the skillet.
5. Simmer the mixture for 10 minutes, stirring occasionally, until flavors are well combined.
6. Taste and adjust seasoning if needed. Garnish with fresh parsley, if desired. Serve warm.
7. Pair with crusty bread or a side of rice to soak up the flavorful sauce.

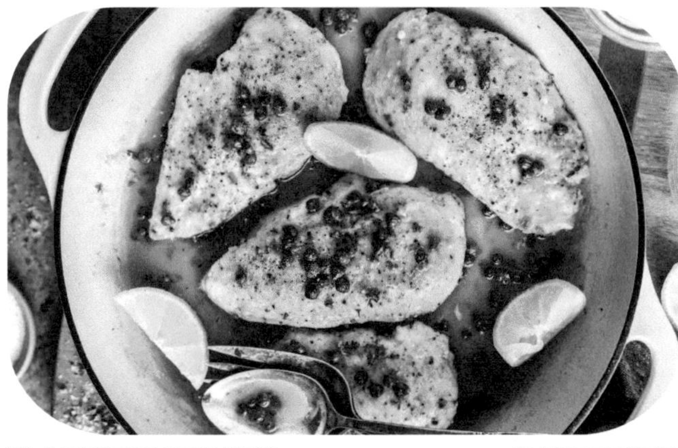

Lemon and Caper Chicken Piccata

PREPARATION TIME: 10 MINUTES

COOKING TIME: 15-20 MINUTES

SERVES: 4

Nutrition Information (Per Serving):
320 Calories / 18g Fat / 6g Carbohydrates / 28g Protein / 500mg Sodium / 1g Sugar

INGREDIENTS:

- 4 boneless, skinless chicken breasts
- 1/4 cup flour (for dredging)
- Salt and pepper to taste
- 3 tablespoons olive oil
- 3 cloves garlic, minced
- 1/2 cup chicken broth
- Juice of 1 lemon
- 2 tablespoons capers, drained
- 2 tablespoons unsalted butter
- Fresh parsley, chopped (for garnish)
- Lemon slices, for serving

DIRECTIONS:

1. Season the chicken breasts with salt and pepper, then dredge them in flour, shaking off any excess.
2. Heat the olive oil in a large skillet over medium-high heat. Cook the chicken for 3-4 minutes on each side until golden and cooked through. Remove the chicken from the skillet and set it aside.
3. In the same skillet, add the minced garlic and cook for about 1 minute until fragrant. Pour in the chicken broth and lemon juice, scraping up any browned bits from the bottom of the skillet. Let it simmer for 2-3 minutes.
4. Stir in the capers and butter, cooking until the butter melts and the sauce is smooth.
5. Return the chicken to the skillet, spooning the sauce over the top. Cook for an additional 8-10 minutes or until the chicken is fully cooked through.
6. Garnish with fresh parsley and serve with your favorite side dish.

Kofta Kebab

PREPARATION TIME: 15 MINUTES

COOKING TIME: 15 MINUTES

SERVES: 4

Nutrition Information (Per Serving):
400 Calories / 24g Fat / 3g Carbohydrates / 28g Protein / 500mg Sodium / 1g Sugar

INGREDIENTS:

- 1 ½ lb ground beef
- 1 small onion, finely grated
- 2 garlic cloves, minced
- 1 ½ cups fresh parsley, chopped
- 2 teaspoons dried oregano
- Salt and pepper, to taste
- 1 egg (optional, for binding)
- 2 tablespoons olive oil (for brushing)

DIRECTIONS:

1. In a large bowl, combine the ground beef, grated onion, minced garlic, chopped parsley, dried oregano, and the egg (if using). Season with a big pinch of salt and pepper. Mix well until all ingredients are evenly combined.
2. Divide the mixture into 8 equal parts. Shape each portion into a cylinder around a metal skewer, pressing firmly to ensure the mixture adheres.
3. Heat 3 tablespoons of olive oil in a griddle pan over medium heat. Once hot, add the kofta kebabs.
4. Cook the kebabs for 8-10 minutes, turning every 1-2 minutes until they are deeply golden and lightly charred on all sides.
5. Serve the kofta kebabs hot, alongside tzatziki and a fresh Greek salad.

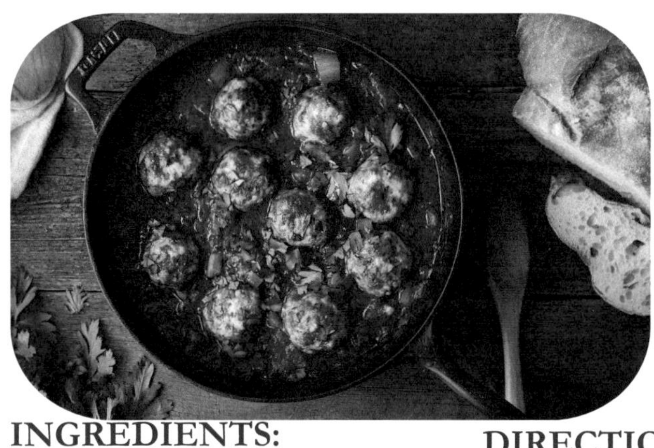

Turkey Meatballs in Tomato Sauce

PREPARATION TIME: 10 MINUTES

COOKING TIME: 10-12 MINUTES

SERVES: 4

Nutrition Information (Per Serving):
250 Calories / 12g Fat / 12g Carbohydrates / 22g Protein / 350mg Sodium / 5g Sugar

INGREDIENTS:

For the Meatballs:

- 1 lb ground turkey
- 1/3 cup breadcrumbs
- 1 egg
- 1 clove garlic, minced
- 1/2 teaspoon oregano
- Salt and pepper

For the Tomato Sauce:

- 1 tablespoon olive oil
- 1 small onion, chopped
- 2 garlic cloves, minced
- 1 can (14 oz) diced tomatoes
- 1/4 cup tomato paste
- 1/2 teaspoon basil
- Salt and pepper

DIRECTIONS:

1. In a large bowl, mix the ground turkey, breadcrumbs, egg, parsley, minced garlic, oregano, cumin, salt, and pepper. Form the mixture into small meatballs (about 1-1.5 inches in diameter).
2. Heat olive oil in a large skillet over medium heat. Add the meatballs and cook for 5-7 minutes, turning occasionally, until browned on all sides. Remove from the skillet and set aside.
3. In the same skillet, add the onion and sauté for 2-3 minutes until softened. Add the garlic and cook for 1 minute until fragrant.
4. Stir in the diced tomatoes, tomato paste, basil, smoked paprika (if using), salt, and pepper. Simmer the sauce for 5 minutes.
5. Return the meatballs to the skillet, covering them with the tomato sauce. Cover and simmer for another 10 minutes, or until the meatballs are fully cooked and flavors meld together.

Moroccan Chicken with Chickpeas

PREPARATION 10 MINUTES

COOKING TIME: 20-25 MINUTES

SERVES: 4

Nutrition Information (Per Serving):
320 Calories / 15g Fat / 2g Carbohydrates / 40g Protein / 350mg Sodium / 1g Sugar

INGREDIENTS:

- 6-8 bone-in, skin-on chicken thighs
- 1 cup canned chickpeas, rinsed
- 1 onion, sliced
- 4 garlic cloves, minced
- 1 cup diced tomatoes
- 2 tablespoons olive oil
- 2 teaspoons ground cumin, cinnamon, turmeric (combined)
- 1/2 teaspoon ground ginger
- Salt and pepper, to taste
- 1 cup chicken broth (or water)
- 1/2 cup raisins (optional)
- Fresh parsley (optional, for garnish)

DIRECTIONS:

1. Heat olive oil in a large pan over medium-high heat. Season the chicken thighs with salt, pepper, and the combined spices. Sear the chicken for 2-3 minutes per side until golden brown. Remove and set aside.
2. In the same pan, sauté the onions for 3 minutes until softened. Add the garlic and cook for 1 minute until fragrant.
3. Add the chickpeas, diced tomatoes, and chicken broth. Stir everything together, then return the chicken to the pan.
4. Cover the pan and simmer on medium heat for 15 minutes, until the chicken is fully cooked and the flavors meld.
5. Taste and adjust seasoning as needed. Garnish with parsley before serving.

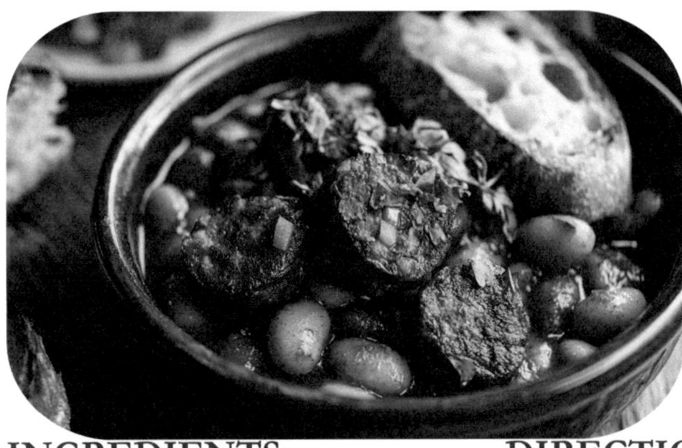

Turkish Beans with Sausage

PREPARATION TIME: 10 MINUTES

COOKING TIME: 20 MINUTES

SERVES: 4

Nutrition Information (Per Serving):
400 Calories / 18g Fat / 30g Carbohydrates / 25g Protein / 800mg Sodium / 6g Sugar

INGREDIENTS:

- 1 tablespoon olive oil
- 8 oz Turkish sausage (sucuk), chorizo, or any similar spiced sausage, sliced
- 1 onion, finely chopped
- 2 garlic cloves, minced
- 2 cups cooked white beans (canned or pre-cooked)
- 1 can (14 oz) diced tomatoes
- 1 tablespoon tomato paste
- 1 teaspoon paprika
- 1/2 teaspoon ground cumin
- 1/2 teaspoon red chili flakes (optional)
- 1 cup chicken or vegetable stock
- Salt and pepper, to taste
- Fresh parsley, chopped (optional, for garnish)

DIRECTIONS:

1. Heat olive oil in a large skillet or pot over medium heat. Add the sliced sausage and cook for 2-3 minutes until browned. Remove and set aside.
2. In the same skillet, add the chopped onion and sauté for 3-4 minutes until softened. Stir in the garlic and cook for 1 minute until fragrant.
3. Stir in the diced tomatoes, tomato paste, paprika, cumin, and chili flakes (if using). Cook for 2-3 minutes, allowing the flavors to meld.
4. Add the cooked beans, browned sausage, and stock to the skillet. Mix well and bring to a gentle simmer. Cook for 10 minutes, stirring occasionally, until the sauce thickens and everything is heated through.
5. Taste and adjust seasoning with salt and pepper as needed. Garnish with chopped parsley and serve warm with crusty bread or rice.

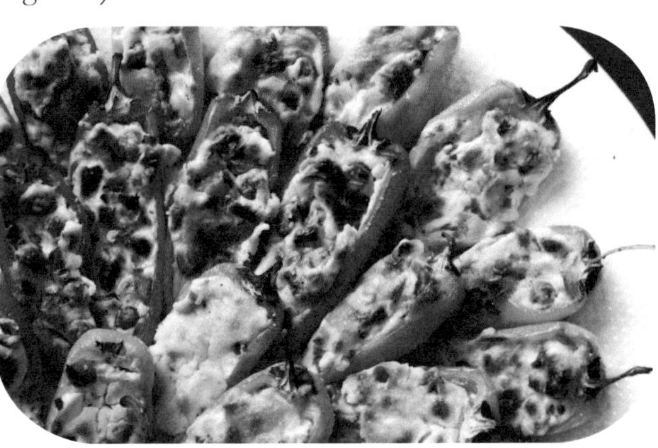

Stuffed Mini Bell Peppers

PREPARATION 10 MINUTES

COOKING TIME: 20-25 MINUTES

SERVES: 4

Nutrition Information (Per Serving):
220 Calories / 15g Fat / 5g Carbohydrates / 16g Protein / 200mg Sodium / 2g Sugar

INGREDIENTS:

- 12 -15 mini bell peppers, halved and seeds removed
- 1/2 lb ground beef or turkey
- 1/4 cup cream cheese, softened
- 1/4 cup feta cheese, crumbled
- 1/4 cup diced onions
- 2 tablespoons olive oil (divided)
- 1 clove garlic, minced
- 1 tablespoon fresh parsley, chopped
- Salt and pepper to taste

DIRECTIONS:

1. Preheat your oven to 375°F (190°C). Line a baking sheet with parchment paper.
2. Heat 1 tablespoon of olive oil in a skillet over medium heat. Add the diced onion and sauté for 2-3 minutes until softened. Add the ground meat and minced garlic, cooking until browned. Season with salt and pepper, then remove from heat and let cool slightly.
3. In a bowl, mix the cooked ground meat, softened cream cheese, crumbled feta, and parsley until well combined.
4. Fill each mini bell pepper half with the beef and cheese mixture, pressing gently to ensure even filling.
5. Arrange the stuffed peppers on the prepared baking sheet and drizzle with the remaining olive oil. Bake for 15 minutes, or until the peppers are tender and the filling is golden.

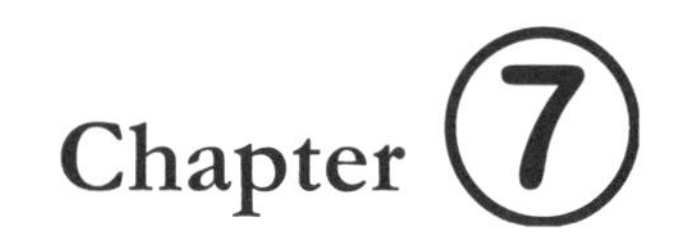

DESSERTS

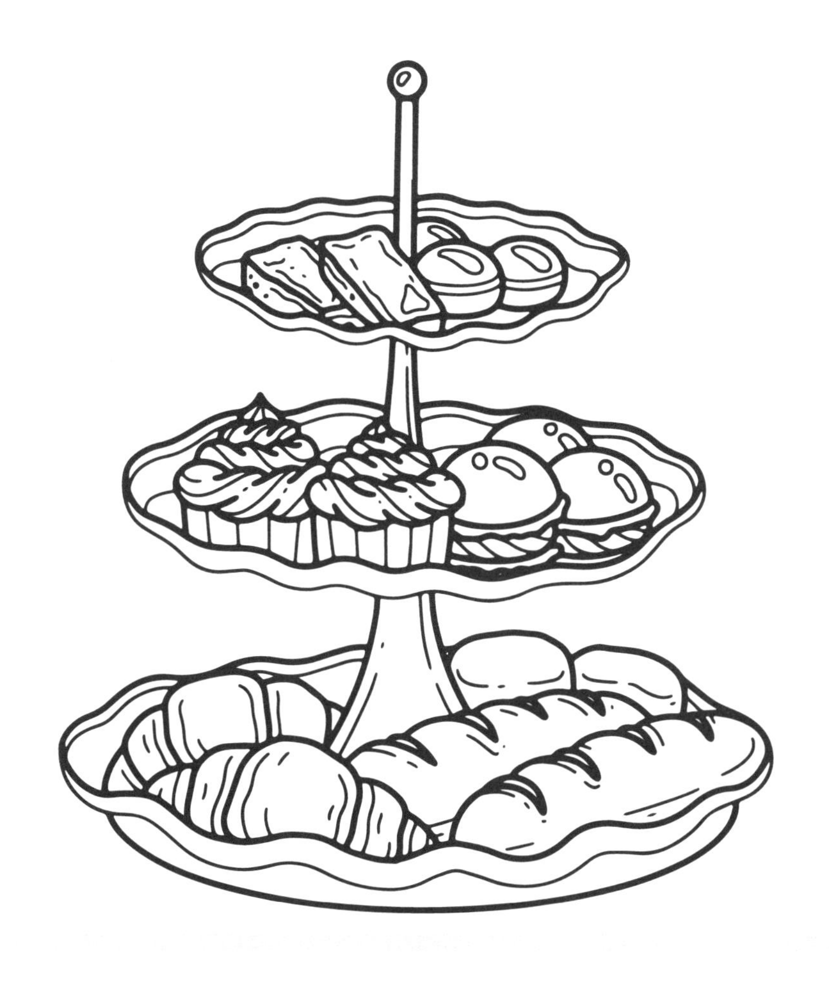

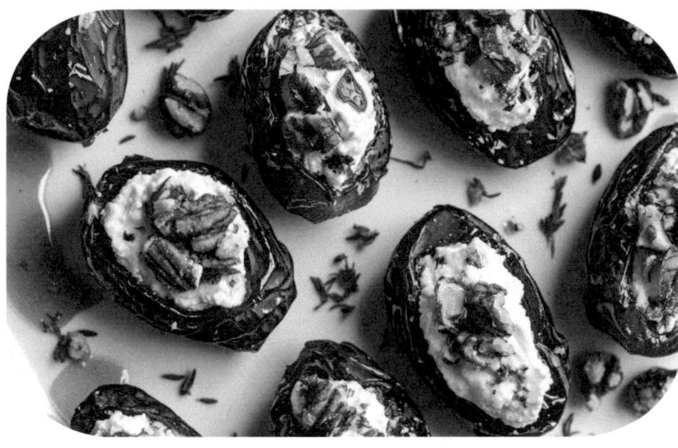

Stuffed Dates with Nuts and Goat Cheese

PREPARATION TIME: 10 MINUTES

COOKING TIME: NONE

SERVES: 4

Nutrition Information (Per Serving):
120 Calories / 6g Fat / 14g Carbohydrates / 3g Protein / 60mg Sodium / 11g Sugar

INGREDIENTS:

- 20 Medjool dates, pitted
- 4 oz goat cheese, softened
- 1/4 cup chopped nuts (such as almonds, walnuts, or pistachios)
- 1 tablespoon honey (optional, for drizzling)
- Fresh herbs (such as thyme or rosemary) for garnish (optional)

DIRECTIONS:

1. Slice each date lengthwise to create an opening, being careful not to cut all the way through.
2. Fill each date with about 1/2 teaspoon of goat cheese.
3. Sprinkle the stuffed dates with chopped nuts.
4. Arrange the dates on a serving platter.
5. If desired, drizzle with honey and garnish with fresh herbs.
6. Serve immediately.

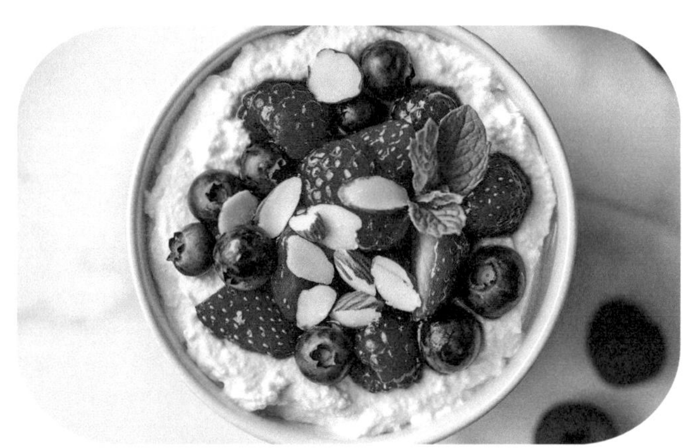

Honey Ricotta with Fresh Berries

PREPARATION TIME: 10 MINUTES

COOKING TIME: NONE

SERVES: 4

Nutrition Information (Per Serving):
220 Calories / 12g Fat / 19g Carbohydrates / 8g Protein / 80mg Sodium / 16g Sugar

INGREDIENTS:

- 1 cup ricotta cheese
- 2 tablespoons honey
- 1 teaspoon vanilla extract
- 1 cup mixed fresh berries (strawberries, blueberries, raspberries)
- 1/4 cup sliced almonds or chopped nuts (optional)
- Fresh mint leaves for garnish (optional)

DIRECTIONS:

1. In a medium bowl, mix the ricotta cheese, honey, and vanilla extract until smooth and creamy.
2. Divide the ricotta mixture among four serving dishes.
3. Top each dish with a generous portion of fresh berries.
4. Sprinkle with sliced almonds or chopped nuts if desired.
5. Garnish with fresh mint leaves for an extra touch of color and flavor.
6. Serve immediately.

TIP: For an added layer of flavor, drizzle a little more honey over the berries just before serving.

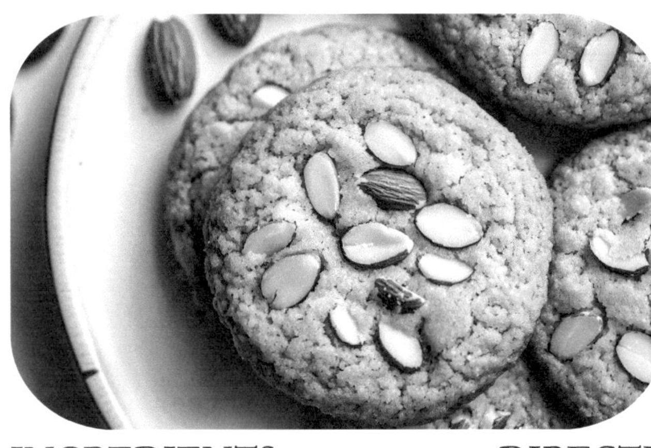

Honey Almond Cookies

PREPARATION TIME: 10 MINUTES

COOKING TIME: 15-20 MINUTES

SERVES: 4 (MAKES ABOUT 15 COOKIES)

Nutrition Information (Per Cookie):
120 Calories / 7g Fat / 12g Carbohydrates / 2g Protein / 50mg Sodium / 8g Sugar

INGREDIENTS:

- 1 1/2 cups almond flour
- 1/4 cup honey
- 1/4 cup unsalted butter, melted
- 1/2 teaspoon vanilla extract
- 1/4 teaspoon almond extract (optional)
- 1/4 teaspoon baking powder
- 1/4 teaspoon salt
- 1/4 cup sliced almonds, for topping

DIRECTIONS:

1. Preheat the oven to 350°F (175°C) and line a baking sheet with parchment paper.
2. In a bowl, mix almond flour, baking powder, and salt. In another bowl, whisk melted butter, honey, vanilla, and almond extract.
3. Combine wet and dry ingredients to form a dough.
4. Roll tablespoon-sized portions of dough into balls, flatten slightly, and place on the baking sheet. Top with sliced almonds.
5. Bake for 15-20 minutes until the edges are golden. Cool on the baking sheet for a few minutes, then transfer to a wire rack to cool completely.

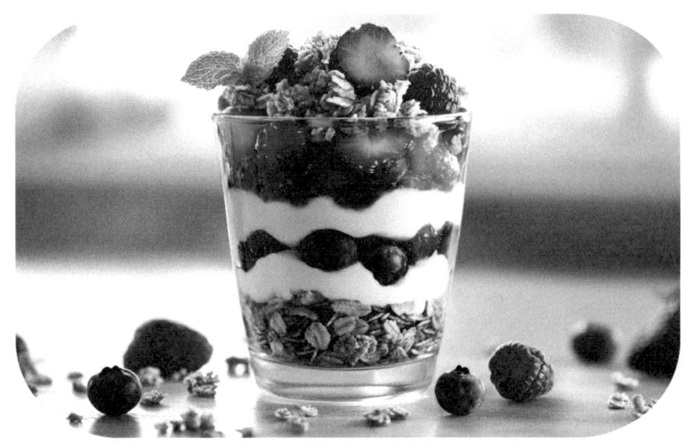

Yogurt and Berry Parfait

PREPARATION TIME: 15 MINUTES

COOKING TIME: NONE

SERVES: 4

Nutrition Information (Per Serving):
180 Calories / 6g Fat / 25g Carbohydrates / 7g Protein / 70mg Sodium / 18g Sugar

INGREDIENTS:

- 2 cups Greek yogurt
- 2 tablespoons honey or maple syrup
- 1 teaspoon vanilla extract
- 2 cups mixed berries (strawberries, blueberries, raspberries)
- 1/2 cup granola
- Fresh mint leaves for garnish (optional)

DIRECTIONS:

1. In a medium bowl, stir together the Greek yogurt, honey, and vanilla extract until smooth and well combined. Taste and adjust the sweetness by adding more honey if desired.
2. Spoon a layer of the yogurt mixture into the bottom of each serving glass or bowl.
3. Top the yogurt with a layer of mixed berries, followed by a sprinkle of granola.
4. Add another layer of yogurt, then more berries and granola.
5. Continue layering until the glasses are full, finishing with berries and a sprinkle of granola on top.
6. Garnish each parfait with fresh mint leaves if desired.

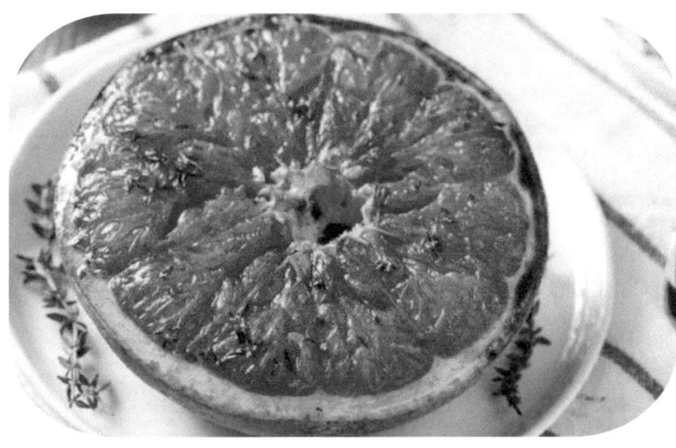

Honey and Cinnamon Baked Grapefruit

PREPARATION TIME: 5 MINUTES

COOKING TIME: 10 -12 MINUTES

SERVES: 4

Nutrition Information (Per Serving):
90 Calories / 2g Fat / 20g Carbohydrates / 1g Protein / 0mg Sodium / 18g Sugar

INGREDIENTS:

- 2 large grapefruits
- 4 tablespoons honey
- 1 teaspoon ground cinnamon
- 1/2 teaspoon vanilla extract (optional)
- Fresh mint leaves for garnish (optional)

DIRECTIONS:

1. Preheat the oven to 375°F (190°C). Line a baking sheet with parchment paper.
2. Cut the grapefruits in half and use a small knife to loosen the segments for easier eating.
3. Place the grapefruit halves on the prepared baking sheet.
4. Drizzle each grapefruit half with 1 tablespoon of honey and sprinkle with ground cinnamon. Add a few drops of vanilla extract if using.
5. Bake in the preheated oven for 10 - 12 minutes, or until the tops are slightly caramelized.
6. Remove from the oven and let cool for a few minutes. Garnish with fresh mint leaves if desired and serve warm.

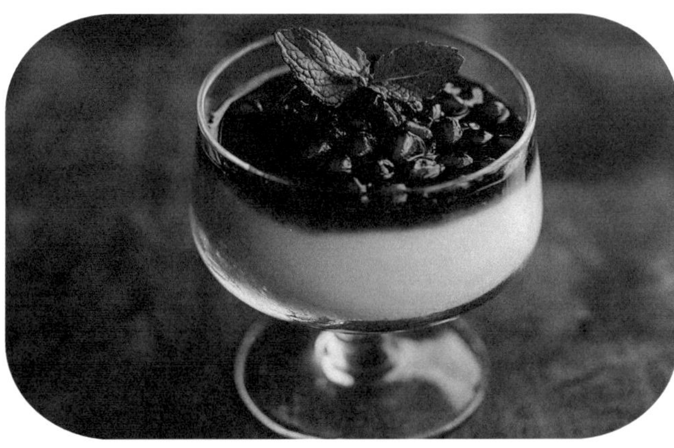

Panna Cotta with Pomegranate Syrup

PREPARATION TIME: 5 MINUTES

COOKING TIME: 10 MINUTES

CHILLING TIME: AT LEAST 15 - 20 MINUTES

SERVES: 4

Nutrition Information (Per Serving):
230 Calories / 14g Fat / 20g Carbohydrates / 4g Protein / 40mg Sodium / 16g Sugar

INGREDIENTS:

- 2 cups heavy cream
- 1/3 cup sugar
- 1 teaspoon vanilla extract
- 1 packet (2 1/4 tsp) unflavored gelatin
- 1/4 cup cold water
- 1 cup pomegranate juice
- 2 tablespoons sugar (for syrup)
- 1/4 cup fresh pomegranate seeds (for garnish, optional)

DIRECTIONS:

1. In a small bowl, sprinkle the gelatin over the cold water and let it sit for 5 minutes to bloom.
2. In a saucepan, heat the heavy cream and sugar over medium heat, stirring until the sugar is dissolved. Do not boil. Remove from heat and stir in the vanilla extract.
3. Add the bloomed gelatin to the warm cream mixture, whisking until completely dissolved.
4. Pour the mixture evenly into 4 ramekins or serving glasses. Let cool slightly, then refrigerate for at least 15 minutes until set.
5. Meanwhile, prepare the pomegranate syrup by heating the pomegranate juice and sugar in a small saucepan over medium heat. Simmer for 5-7 minutes until slightly thickened, then let it cool.
6. To serve, drizzle the pomegranate syrup over the chilled panna cotta and garnish with pomegranate seeds if desired.

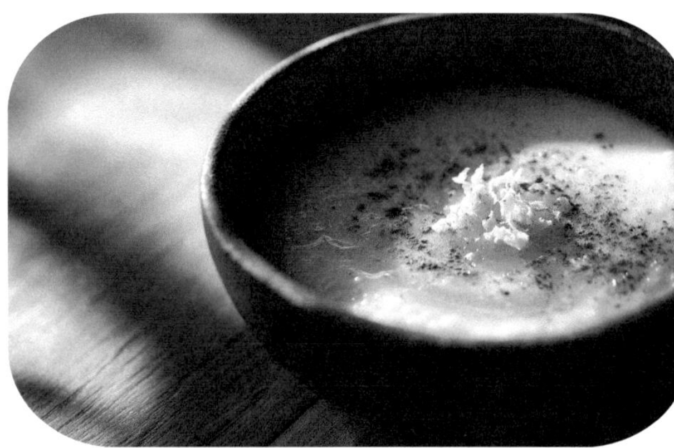

Rizogalo (Mediterranean Rice Pudding)

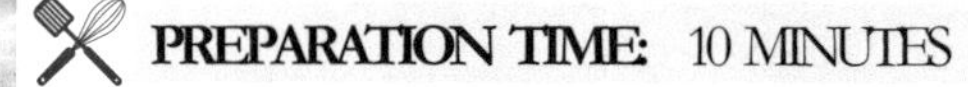

PREPARATION TIME: 10 MINUTES

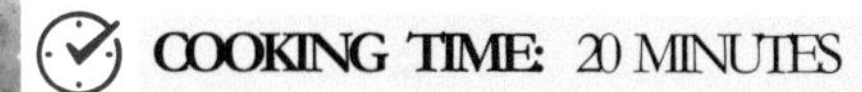

COOKING TIME: 20 MINUTES

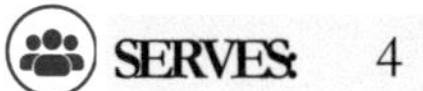

SERVES: 4

Nutrition Information (Per Serving):
200 Calories / 5g Fat / 35g Carbohydrates / 5g Protein / 60mg Sodium / 12g Sugar

INGREDIENTS:

- 1/2 cup short-grain rice (e.g., Arborio or pudding rice)
- 2 cups milk (whole or 2%)
- 1/2 cup water
- 1/4 cup sugar
- 1 teaspoon vanilla extract
- Zest of 1 lemon
- 1/2 teaspoon ground cinnamon (for garnish)

DIRECTIONS:

1. In a medium saucepan, combine the rice, water, and half of the milk. Bring to a gentle simmer over medium heat, stirring occasionally to prevent sticking. Cook until the rice absorbs most of the liquid, about 10 minutes.
2. Gradually add the remaining milk, sugar, and lemon zest, stirring frequently. Continue simmering for another 12-15 minutes, or until the rice is tender and the pudding has thickened to your desired consistency.
3. Remove the saucepan from heat and stir in the vanilla extract. Taste and adjust sweetness if needed.
4. Spoon the rice pudding into serving bowls while warm. Sprinkle with ground cinnamon and serve immediately, or let it cool and refrigerate for a chilled version.

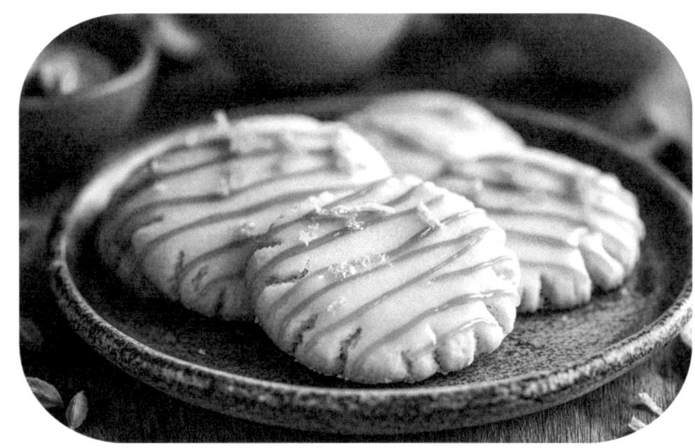

Orange Cardamom Shortbread

PREPARATION TIME: 10 MINUTES

COOKING TIME: 20-25 MINUTES

SERVES: 4 (MAKES ABOUT 12 COOKIES)

Nutrition Information (Per Serving):
180 Calories / 9g Fat / 20g Carbohydrates / 2g Protein / 60mg Sodium / 8g Sugar

INGREDIENTS:

- 1 cup all-purpose flour
- 1/4 cup powdered sugar
- 1/2 cup unsalted butter, softened
- Zest of 1 orange
- 1/2 teaspoon ground cardamom
- A pinch of salt
- Optional: Orange glaze (1/2 cup powdered sugar + 1 tablespoon orange juice)

DIRECTIONS:

1. Preheat your oven to 350°F (175°C). Line a baking sheet with parchment paper.
2. In a mixing bowl, cream together the butter, powdered sugar, and orange zest until smooth and fluffy. Add the flour, cardamom, and salt. Mix until the dough comes together.
3. Roll the dough into small balls (about 1 inch) and flatten slightly with your palm or the back of a fork. Place the cookies on the prepared baking sheet, spacing them about 1 inch apart.
4. Bake for 15-18 minutes, or until the edges are lightly golden. Remove from the oven and let the cookies cool on the baking sheet for 5 minutes before transferring them to a wire rack to cool completely.
5. Optional Glaze:If desired, mix the powdered sugar and orange juice to create a glaze. Drizzle over the cooled cookies for extra sweetness and orange flavor.

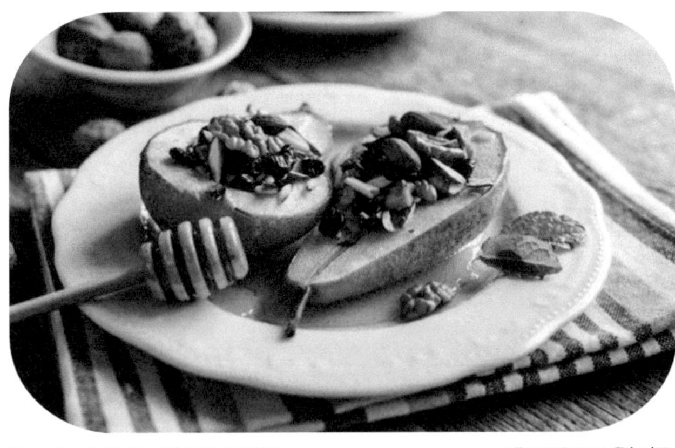

Baked Pears with Honey

PREPARATION TIME: 10 MINUTES

COOKING TIME: 20-25 MINUTES

SERVES: 4

Nutrition Information (Per Serving):
180 Calories / 7g Fat / 28g Carbohydrates / 2g Protein / 15mg Sodium / 18g Sugar

INGREDIENTS:

- 4 ripe pears, halved and cored
- 2 tablespoons honey
- 1 teaspoon cinnamon
- 1/4 cup walnuts and raisin, chopped (optional, for garnish)
- 1 tablespoon butter, melted

DIRECTIONS:

1. Preheat your oven to 375°F (190°C). Line a baking dish with parchment paper or lightly grease it.
2. Arrange the halved and cored pears in the baking dish with the cut side facing up.
3. Drizzle each pear half with honey, sprinkle with cinnamon, and brush lightly with the melted butter.
4. Bake in the preheated oven for 20-25 minutes, or until the pears are tender and slightly caramelized.
5. Garnish the baked pears with chopped walnuts if desired, and serve warm.

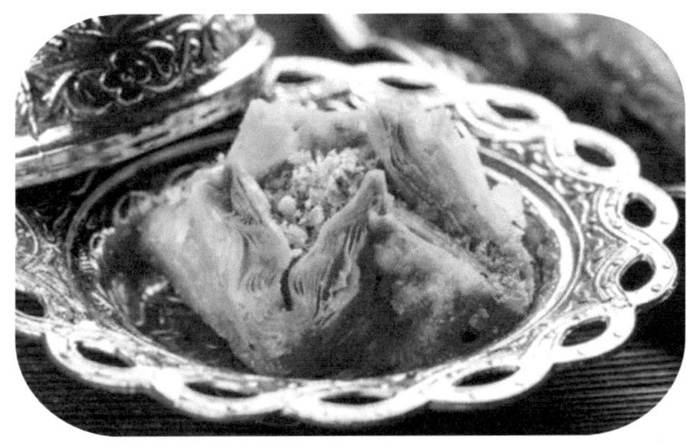

Baklava Bites

PREPARATION TIME: 10 MINUTES

COOKING TIME: 20-25 MINUTES

SERVES: 4

Nutrition Information (Per Serving):
200 Calories / 9g Fat / 12g Carbohydrates / 2g Protein / 50mg Sodium / 8g Sugar

INGREDIENTS:

- 1 sheet phyllo dough, thawed
- 1/2 cup chopped nuts (such as almonds, walnuts, or pistachios)
- 1/4 cup honey
- 1/4 cup butter, melted
- 1/2 teaspoon cinnamon

DIRECTIONS:

1. Preheat your oven to 350°F (175°C). Grease a mini muffin tin or line it with paper liners.
2. Cut the phyllo dough into small squares that fit into the mini muffin tin cups. Layer 3-4 squares of phyllo in each cup, brushing each layer lightly with melted butter.
3. In a bowl, mix the chopped nuts with cinnamon. Spoon a small amount of the nut mixture into each phyllo cup.
4. Drizzle a little honey over each filled cup. Bake in the preheated oven for 20-25 minutes, or until the phyllo is golden brown and crispy.
5. Allow the baklava bites to cool slightly before removing them from the muffin tin. Drizzle with additional honey if desired and serve.

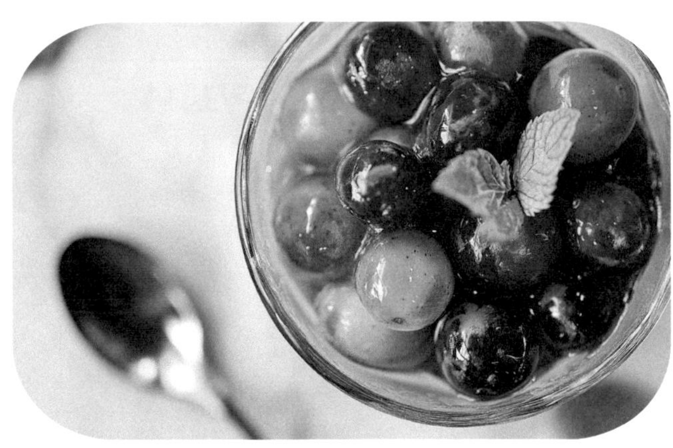

Grapes in Muscat Syrup

PREPARATION TIME: 5 MINUTES

COOKING TIME: 5 MINUTES

CHILLING TIME: AT LEAST 20 - 25 MINUTES

SERVES: 4

Nutrition Information (Per Serving):
120 Calories / 0g Fat / 28g Carbohydrates / 1g Protein / 0mg Sodium / 26g Sugar

INGREDIENTS:

- 2 cups seedless grapes (red or green)
- 1/2 cup Muscat wine (or any sweet dessert wine)
- 2 tablespoons honey
- 1 teaspoon lemon juice
- 1/2 teaspoon vanilla extract
- Fresh mint leaves for garnish (optional)

DIRECTIONS:

1. In a small saucepan, combine the Muscat wine, honey, lemon juice, and vanilla extract.
2. Bring the mixture to a gentle simmer over low heat, stirring until the honey is fully dissolved.
3. Remove from heat and let the syrup cool to room temperature.
4. Place the grapes in a serving bowl or divide them into individual dessert glasses.
5. Pour the cooled syrup over the grapes, making sure they are well coated.
6. Cover and refrigerate for at least 1 hour to allow the flavors to meld.
7. Serve the chilled grapes in their syrup, garnished with fresh mint leaves if desired.

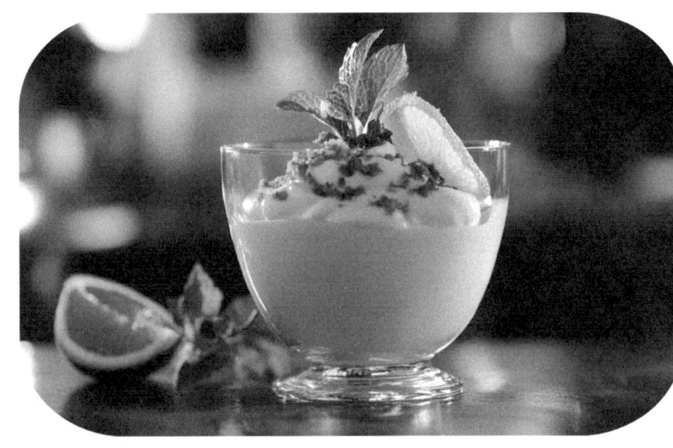

Yogurt and Orange Zest Mousse

PREPARATION TIME: 10 MINUTES

COOKING TIME: NONE

CHILLING TIME: AT LEAST 20 - 25 MINUTES

SERVES: 4

Nutrition Information (Per Serving):
180 Calories / 9g Fat / 12g Carbohydrates / 6g Protein / 50mg Sodium / 8g Sugar

INGREDIENTS:

- 2 cups plain Greek yogurt
- 1 cup heavy cream
- 6 tablespoons honey or maple syrup
- Zest of 2 oranges
- 1 teaspoon vanilla extract
- Orange slices or mint leaves for garnish (optional)

DIRECTIONS:

1. In a large mixing bowl, whisk together the Greek yogurt, honey (or maple syrup), orange zest, and vanilla extract until smooth.
2. In a separate bowl, whip the heavy cream until soft peaks form.
3. Gently fold the whipped cream into the yogurt mixture to maintain its airy texture.
4. Divide the mousse evenly into 4 serving glasses or bowls. Chill in the refrigerator for at least 20 minutes to allow the flavors to meld.
5. Garnish with orange slices or mint leaves, if desired, and serve cold for a refreshing Mediterranean dessert.

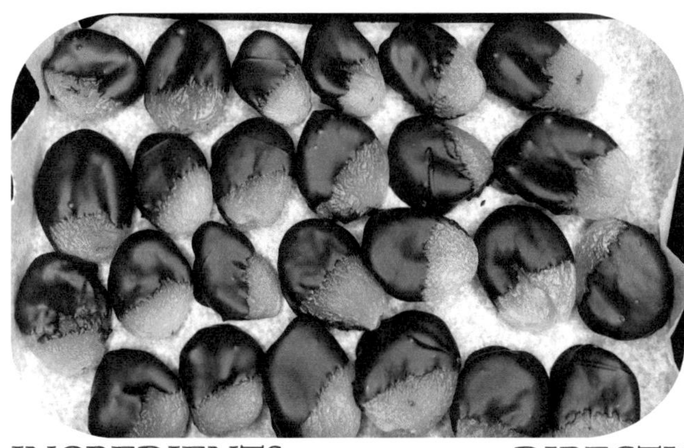

Chocolate-Dipped Apricots

PREPARATION TIME: 5 MINUTES

COOKING TIME: 10 MINUTES

CHILLING TIME: AT LEAST 15 - 20 MINUTES

SERVES: 24 pieces

Nutrition Information (per piece):
60 Calories / 3g Fat / 7g Carbohydrates / 1g Protein / 10mg Sodium / 6g Sugar

INGREDIENTS:

- 24 dried apricots
- 1 cup dark chocolate chips (or chocolate bar, chopped)
- 1 tablespoon coconut oil
- Sea salt (optional, for a touch of flavor)

DIRECTIONS:

1. In a microwave-safe bowl, combine the dark chocolate chips and coconut oil. Microwave in 30-second intervals, stirring in between, until the chocolate is fully melted and smooth.
2. Dip each dried apricot halfway into the melted chocolate, allowing the excess to drip off. Place the dipped apricots on a parchment-lined baking sheet.
3. Sprinkle the chocolate-dipped apricots with a light sprinkle of sea salt, if desired.
4. Let the apricots cool at room temperature or place them in the refrigerator for 15-20 minutes until the chocolate is set.
5. Enjoy the chocolate-dipped apricots as a sweet snack or dessert.

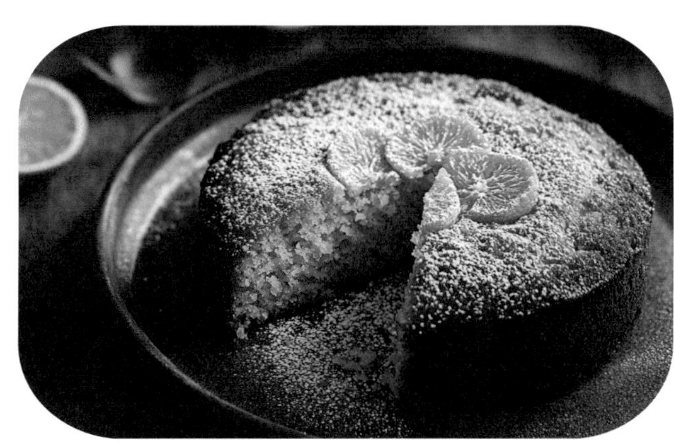

Quick Orange and Almond Cake

PREPARATION TIME: 5 MINUTES

COOKING TIME: 25 MINUTES

SERVES: 4

Nutrition Information (Per Serving):
200 Calories / 12g Fat / 15g Carbohydrates / 6g Protein / 80mg Sodium / 8g Sugar

INGREDIENTS:

- 1 cup almond flour
- 2 large eggs
- 1/3 cup honey or maple syrup
- Zest of 1 orange
- 2 tablespoons fresh orange juice
- 1/2 teaspoon baking powder
- 1/2 teaspoon vanilla extract
- A pinch of salt
- Powdered sugar or orange slices for garnish (optional)

DIRECTIONS:

1. Preheat your oven to 350°F (175°C). Grease a small 6-inch cake pan or line it with parchment paper.
2. In a mixing bowl, whisk together the eggs, honey (or maple syrup), orange zest, orange juice, and vanilla extract until smooth.
3. Add the almond flour, baking powder, and a pinch of salt to the wet ingredients. Mix gently until well combined.
4. Pour the batter into the prepared cake pan and spread it evenly.
5. Bake for 20-25 minutes, or until the cake is golden and a toothpick inserted into the center comes out clean.
6. Allow the cake to cool for 5 minutes before transferring it to a wire rack to cool completely.
7. Garnish with a light dusting of powdered sugar or fresh orange slices, if desired. Slice and serve.

Chapter 8

REFRESHERS

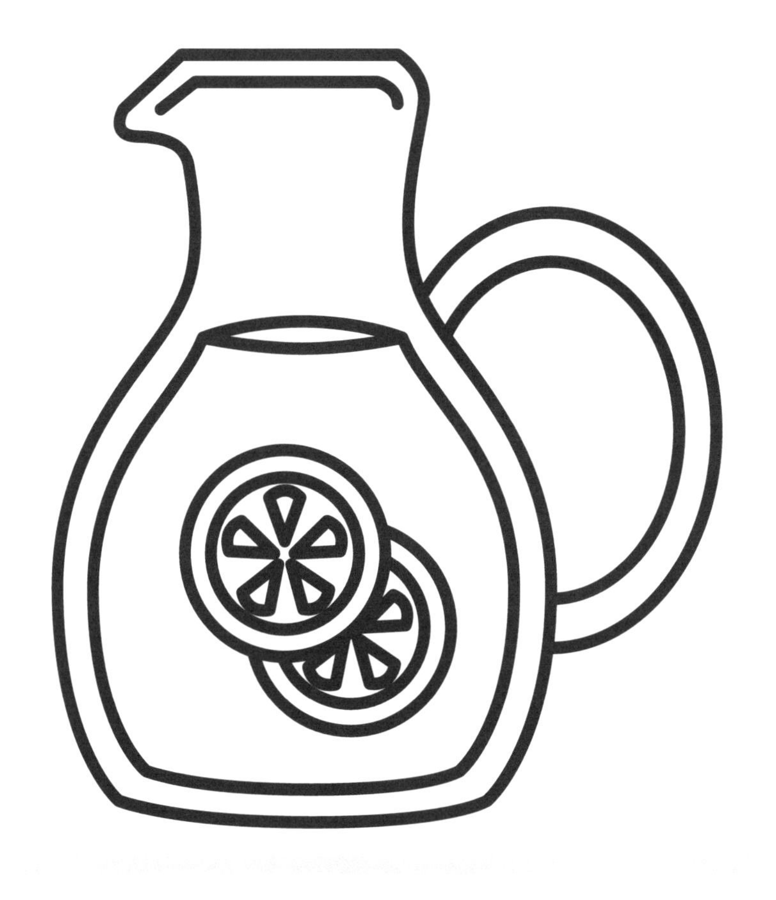

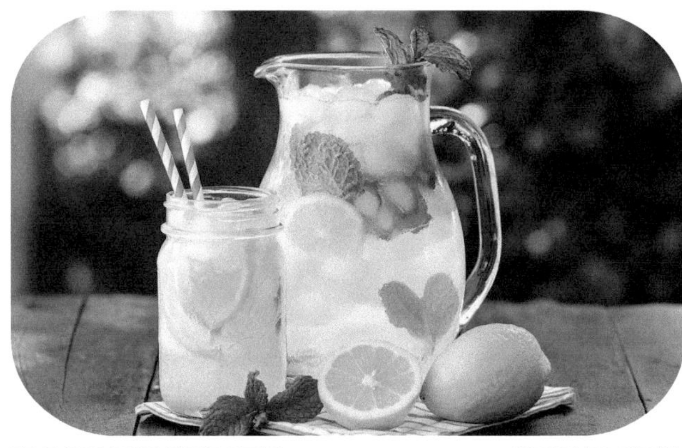

Lemon Mint Cooler

PREPARATION TIME: 10 MINUTES

COOKING TIME: NONE

CHILLING TIME: 20-25 MINUTES

SERVES: 6-8 GLASSES

Nutrition Information (Per Serving):
50 Calories / 0g Fat / 13g Carbohydrates / 0g Protein / 4mg Sodium / 12g Sugar

INGREDIENTS:

- 3/4 cup fresh lemon juice (about 4-6 lemons)
- 1/3 cup fresh mint leaves
- 1/3 cup sugar (adjust to taste)
- 6 cups cold water
- Ice cubes (as needed)

DIRECTIONS:

1. In a large pitcher or jar, mix the fresh lemon juice and sugar, stirring until the sugar dissolves completely.
2. Add the fresh mint leaves and gently muddle them to release their flavor.
3. Pour in the cold water and stir well to combine.
4. Add ice cubes and chill in the refrigerator for at least 20-25 minutes before serving.
5. Serve in individual glasses with extra ice and a sprig of mint for garnish.

TIP: Add lemon slices and crushed mint to the pitcher for extra flavor.

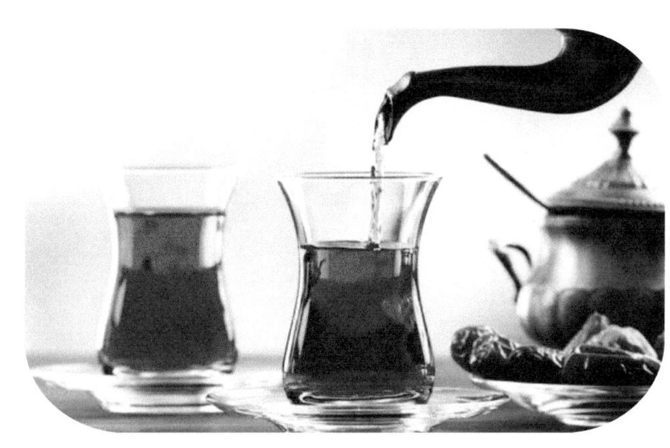

Traditional Hot Turkish Tea with Lemon

PREPARATION TIME: 10 MINUTES

COOKING TIME: NONE

BREWING TIME: 15-20 MINUTES

SERVES: 4 CUPS

Nutrition Information (Per Cup):
5 Calories / 0g Fat / 1g Carbohydrates / 0g Protein / 0mg Sodium / 1g Sugar (without added sugar)

INGREDIENTS:

- 4 cups of brewed black tea (strong)
- Juice of 1 lemon
- 3 tablespoons honey (adjust to taste)
- 1/2 lemon, sliced

DIRECTIONS:

1. In a medium saucepan, boil 4 cups of water.
2. Add 3 tablespoons of loose black tea leaves to a small teapot.
3. Pour 1 cup of boiling water into the teapot to bloom the tea leaves.
4. Add the remaining water to the teapot, then place it on the saucepan and let it simmer for 15-20 minutes.
5. After simmering, pour the concentrated tea into each Turkish tea glass or regular cup.
6. Add the juice of 1 lemon and a lemon slice to each glass.
7. Dilute with hot water to your desired strength.
8. Serve with sugar on the side for individual taste.

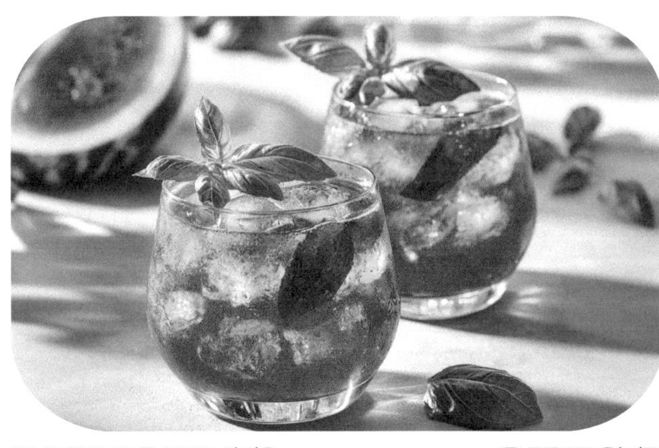

Watermelon Basil Cooler

PREPARATION TIME: 10 MINUTES

COOKING TIME: NONE

SERVES: 4 GLASSES

Nutrition Information (Per Glass):
50 Calories / 0g Fat / 12g Carbohydrates / 1g Protein / 5mg Sodium / 10g Sugar

INGREDIENTS:

- 4 cups fresh watermelon juice (blended watermelon)
- 1/4 cup fresh basil leaves
- Juice of 1 lime
- 1 cup sparkling water
- Ice cubes (as needed)

DIRECTIONS:

1. In a blender, blend the watermelon pieces until smooth. Strain the juice if desired to remove the pulp.
2. In a large pitcher, combine the watermelon juice, lime juice, and fresh basil leaves.
3. Gently muddle the basil leaves with a spoon to release their aroma and flavor.
4. Add the sparkling water and stir well.
5. Fill each glass with ice cubes and pour the Watermelon Basil Cooler over the ice.
6. Garnish with a basil leaf or a small slice of watermelon on the rim.

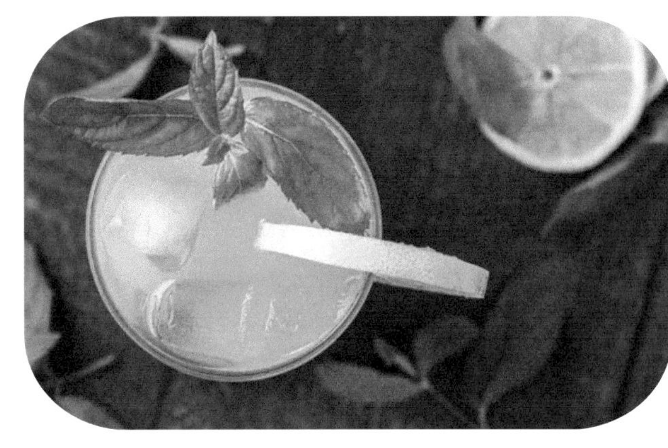

Limoncello Spritz

PREPARATION TIME: 5 MINUTES

COOKING TIME: NONE

SERVES: 4 GLASSES

Nutrition Information (Per Serving):
120 Calories / 0g Fat / 14g Carbohydrates / 0g Protein / 10mg Sodium / 10g Sugar

INGREDIENTS:

- 1 cup Limoncello
- 2 cups soda water or sparkling water
- 1/2 cup Prosecco (optional for extra fizz)
- Ice cubes (as needed)
- Lemon slices and fresh mint leaves (for garnish)

DIRECTIONS:

1. Fill each glass with ice cubes.
2. Pour 1/4 cup of Limoncello into each glass.
3. Add 1/2 cup of soda water or sparkling water to each glass.
4. If desired, top with a splash of Prosecco for an extra touch of bubbles.
5. Stir gently to combine.
6. Garnish with a lemon slice and a sprig of fresh mint for a refreshing finish.
7. Serve immediately and enjoy the light, citrusy taste.

TIP: For a sweeter twist, add a splash of simple syrup or a few fresh berries to the glass before mixing the spritz.

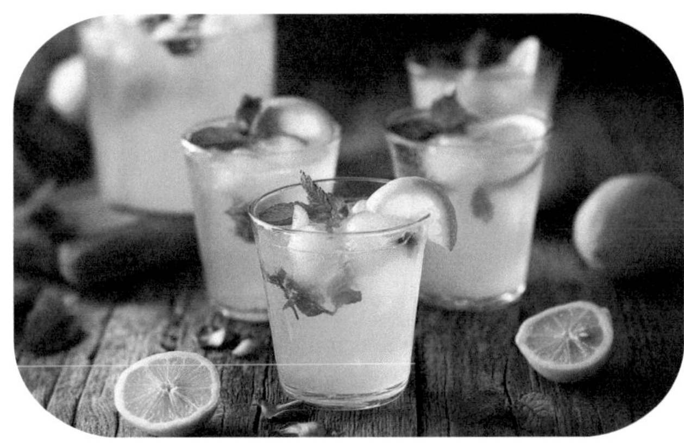

Rosewater Lemonade

 **PREPARATION TIME:** 10 MINUTES

 **COOKING TIME:** NONE

SERVES: 6-8 GLASSES

Nutrition Information (Per Glass):
60 Calories / 0g Fat / 16g Carbohydrates / 0g Protein / 5mg Sodium / 15g Sugar

INGREDIENTS:

- 1 1/2 cups fresh lemon juice (about 8-10 lemons)
- 1/2 cup sugar (adjust to taste)
- 8 cups cold water
- 2 tablespoons rosewater
- Ice cubes (as needed)
- Lemon slices and fresh mint leaves for
garnish (optional)

DIRECTIONS:

1. In a large pitcher, combine the fresh lemon juice and sugar, stirring until the sugar is fully dissolved.
2. Add the rosewater and cold water, then stir well to blend all the ingredients.
3. Fill each glass with ice cubes, and pour the rosewater lemonade mixture over the ice.
4. Garnish with lemon slices and fresh mint leaves for an extra touch of flavor and color.
5. Serve immediately for a refreshing, aromatic drink.

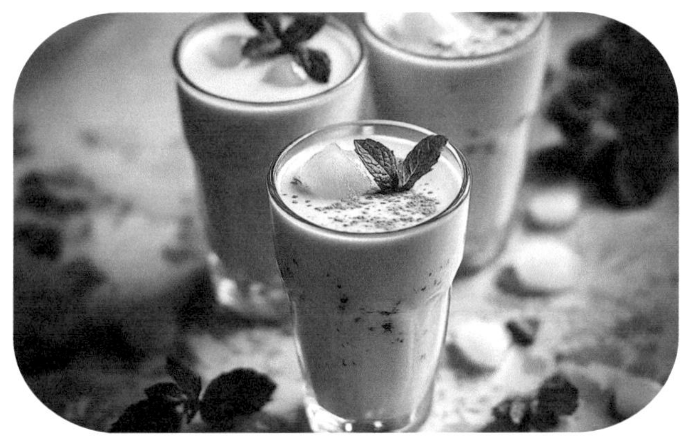

Minty Yogurt Lassi

 **PREPARATION TIME:** 5 MINUTES

 **COOKING TIME:** NONE

SERVES: 4 GLASSES

Nutrition Information (Per Serving):
90 Calories / 3g Fat / 9g Carbohydrates / 6g Protein / 150mg Sodium / 6g Sugar

INGREDIENTS:

- 2 cups Greek yogurt
- 1 cup cold water
- 1/4 cup fresh mint leaves
- 1/2 teaspoon salt
- Ice cubes (as needed)

DIRECTIONS:

1. In a blender, combine the Greek yogurt, cold water, fresh mint leaves, and salt.
2. Blend until the mixture is smooth and frothy.
3. Fill each glass with ice cubes, then pour the lassi over the ice.
4. Garnish with a few mint leaves on top for extra freshness.
5. Serve immediately and enjoy the cool, refreshing taste.

TIP: For an extra burst of flavor, chill the mint leaves before blending to enhance the minty freshness in your lassi.

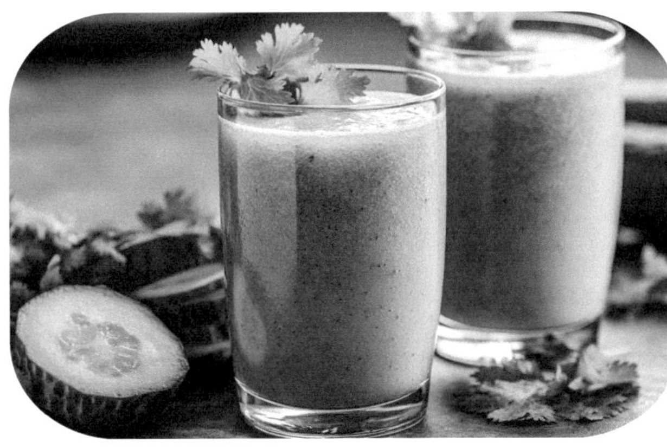

Cucumber Limeade

 **PREPARATION TIME:** 5 MINUTES

 **COOKING TIME:** 5 MINUTES

 **SERVES:** 4 GLASSES

Nutrition Information (Per Glass):
40 Calories / 0g Fat / 10g Carbohydrates / 0g Protein / 2mg Sodium / 8g Sugar.

INGREDIENTS:

- 2 small cucumbers, peeled and chopped
- Juice of 4 limes
- 2 tablespoons honey or sugar (adjust to taste)
- 4 cups cold water
- Ice cubes (as needed)
- Fresh mint leaves (optional, for garnish)

DIRECTIONS:

1. In a blender, combine the chopped cucumbers, lime juice, and honey or sugar. Blend until smooth.
2. Strain the mixture through a fine sieve into a pitcher, discarding the pulp.
3. Stir in the cold water until well combined.
4. Fill four glasses with ice cubes, then pour the cucumber limeade over the ice.
5. Garnish with fresh mint leaves, if desired, and serve immediately.

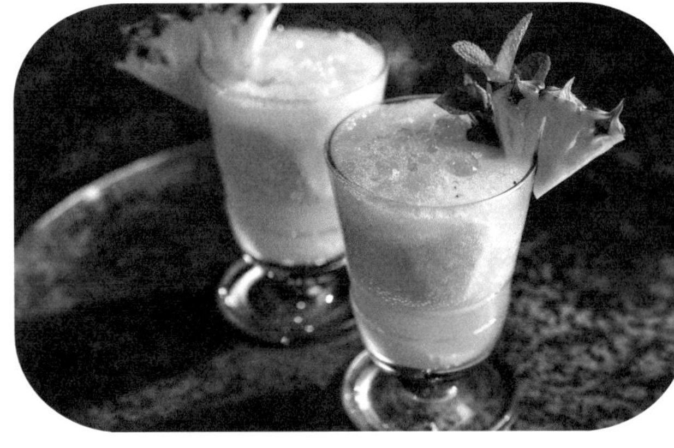

Pineapple Ginger Fizz

 **PREPARATION TIME:** 5 MINUTES

 **COOKING TIME:** NONE

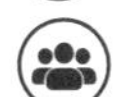 **SERVES:** 4 GLASSES

Nutrition Information (Per Serving):
80 Calories / 0g Fat / 20g Carbohydrates / 1g Protein / 5mg Sodium / 16g Sugar

INGREDIENTS:

- 2 cups pineapple juice (fresh or canned)
- 2 tablespoons fresh ginger, grated
- 2 cups sparkling water or soda water
- Juice of 2 limes
- Ice cubes (as needed)
- Pineapple wedges and mint leaves (for garnish, optional)

DIRECTIONS:

1. In a small bowl, mix the pineapple juice and grated ginger. Let it sit for 5 minutes to infuse the ginger flavor into the juice.
2. Strain the pineapple-ginger mixture into a pitcher, pressing the ginger to extract as much juice as possible.
3. Add the lime juice and stir well.
4. Fill four glasses with ice cubes, then top with sparkling water.
5. Garnish with pineapple wedges and mint leaves, if desired.
6. Serve immediately and enjoy the refreshing, zesty fizz!

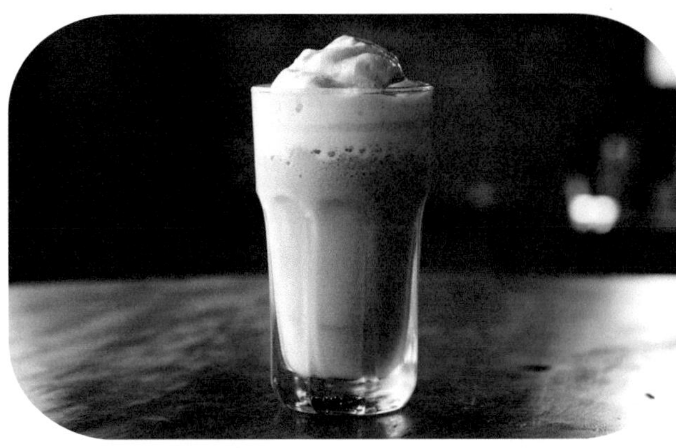

Iced Greek Frappe

PREPARATION TIME: 10 MINUTES

COOKING TIME: NONE

SERVES: 4 GLASSES

Nutrition Information (Per Glass):
40 Calories / 0g Fat / 9g Carbohydrates / 1g Protein / 10mg Sodium / 8g Sugar

INGREDIENTS:

- 1/3 cup instant coffee
- 1 cup cold water
- 1/4 cup sugar (optional, adjust to taste)
- 1 cup milk (optional)
- Ice cubes (as needed)

DIRECTIONS:

1. In a shaker or blender, combine the instant coffee, cold water, and sugar.
2. Blend or shake vigorously for about 20-30 seconds, or until a thick foam forms.
3. Pour the coffee mixture into a pitcher filled with ice cubes.
4. Add milk to taste, or leave it black for a stronger coffee flavor.
5. Stir well before serving, and pour into individual glasses filled with ice if desired.

TIP: For an even creamier texture, blend the frappe with a small scoop of vanilla ice cream or a splash of evaporated milk before serving.

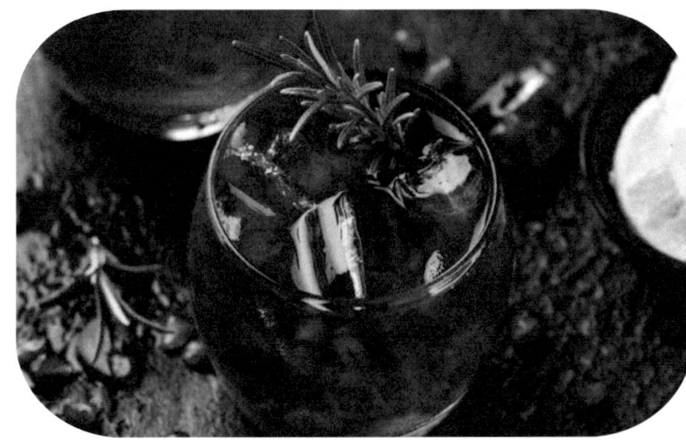

Pomegranate Spritzer

PREPARATION TIME: 5 MINUTES

COOKING TIME: NONE

SERVES: 4 GLASSES

Nutrition Information (Per Serving):
50 Calories / 0g Fat / 13g Carbohydrates / 0g Protein / 5mg Sodium / 12g Sugar

INGREDIENTS:

- 2 cups pomegranate juice
- 2 cups sparkling water
- Juice of 1 lime
- Ice cubes (as needed)
- Fresh rosemary for garnish (optional)

DIRECTIONS:

1. In a large pitcher, combine the pomegranate juice and lime juice.
2. Add the sparkling water and stir gently to mix.
3. Fill each glass with ice cubes, then pour the pomegranate mixture over the ice.
4. Garnish each glass with fresh rosemary for a refreshing finish, if desired.
5. Serve immediately to enjoy its bubbly, tart flavor.

TIP: For a touch of elegance, add a few pomegranate seeds to each glass before serving to enhance the flavor and appearance.

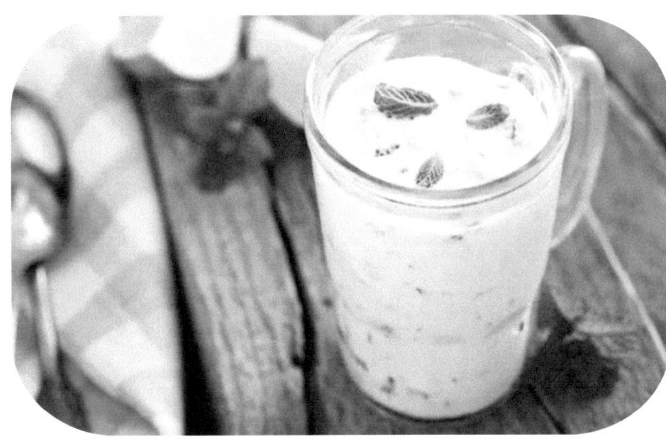

Ayran (Cucumber Yogurt Drink)

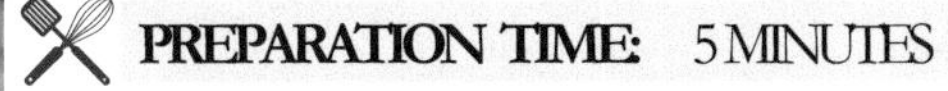

PREPARATION TIME: 5 MINUTES

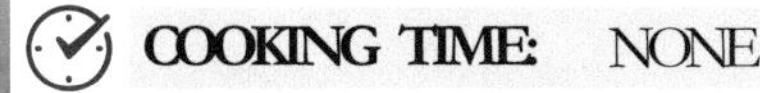

COOKING TIME: NONE

SERVES: 4 GLASSES

Nutrition Information (Per Glass):
70 Calories / 2g Fat / 6g Carbohydrates / 5g Protein / 200mg Sodium / 5g Sugar

INGREDIENTS:

- 2 cups Greek yogurt
- 1 cup cold water
- 1 small cucumber, finely grated or chopped
- 1/2 teaspoon salt
- Ice cubes (as needed)
- Mint leaves for garnish (optional)

DIRECTIONS:

1. In a blender, combine the Greek yogurt, cold water, and salt.
2. Add the grated cucumber and blend until smooth and well combined.
3. Fill four glasses with ice cubes, then pour the Ayran over the ice.
4. Stir well and serve immediately, garnished with a few fresh mint leaves if desired.

TIP: Chill the yogurt and cucumber in the refrigerator before blending to make your Ayran extra cold and refreshing.

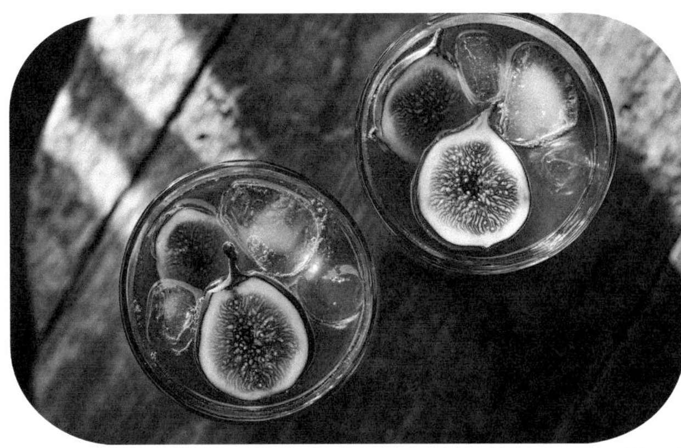

Fig and Honey Iced Tea

PREPARATION TIME: 5 MINUTES

COOKING TIME: NONE

CHILLING TIME: 25 MINUTES

SERVES: 4 GLASSES

Nutrition Information (Per Glass):60 Calories/0g Fat/16g Carbohydrates/0g Protein/5mg Sodium/15g Sugar

INGREDIENTS:

- 4 cups water
- 4 black tea bags
- 4 fresh figs, sliced
- 3 tablespoons honey (adjust to taste)
- Ice cubes (as needed)

DIRECTIONS:

1. Boil the water in a saucepan, then remove from heat and add the black tea bags. Let them steep for about 5 minutes.
2. Remove the tea bags and stir in the honey until fully dissolved.
3. Add the sliced figs to the warm tea and let it cool to room temperature.
4. Once cooled, place the tea in the refrigerator to chill for at least 25 minutes.
5. Fill four glasses with ice cubes, then pour the fig-infused tea over the ice.
6. Garnish with additional fig slices or a sprig of mint for extra flavor.

TIP: For a stronger fig flavor, gently muddle the figs in the tea before chilling to release more of their natural sweetness.

Cooking Measurements & Kitchen Conversions

Dry Measurements Conversion Chart

Teaspoons	Tablespoons	Cups
3 tsp	1 tbsp	1/16 c
6 tsp	2 tbsp	1/8 c
12 tsp	4 tbsp	1/4 c
24 tsp	8 tbsp	1/2 c
36 tsp	12 tbsp	3/4 c
48 tsp	16 tbsp	1 c

Liquid Measurements Conversion Chart

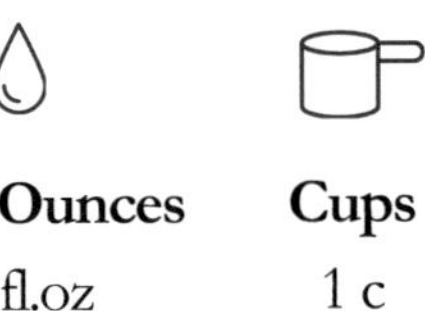

Fluid Ounces	Cups	Pints	Quarts	Gallons
8 fl.oz	1 c	1/2 pt	1/4 qt	1/16 gal
16 fl.oz	2 c	1 pt	1/2 qt	1/8 gal
32 fl.oz	4 c	2 pt	1 qt	1/4 gal
64 fl.oz	8 c	4 pt	2 qt	1/2 gal
128 fl.oz	16 c	8 pt	4 qt	1 gal

Liquid Measurements (Volume)

Standard	Metric
1/5 tsp	1 ml
1 tsp	5 ml
1 tbsp	15 ml
1 c (8 fl.oz)	240 ml
34 fl.oz	1 liter

Dry Measurements (Weight)

Standard	Metric
.035 oz	1 g
3.5 oz	100 g
17.7 oz (1.1 lb)	500 g
35 oz	1 kg

US to Metric Conversions

Standard	Metric
1/5 tsp	1 ml
1 tsp	5 ml
1 tbsp	15 ml
1 fl. oz	30 ml
1 c	237 ml
1 pt	473 ml
1 qt	.95 liter
1 gal	3.8 liters
1 oz	28 g
1 lb	454 g

Oven Temperatures Conversion

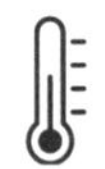

Fahrenheit	Celsius
250 °F	120 °C
320 °F	160 °C
350 °F	180 °C
375 °F	190 °C
400 °F	205 °C
425 °F	220 °C

1 Cup

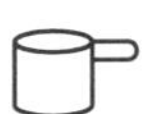

1 cup = 8 fluid ounces
1 cup = 16 tablespoons
1 cup = 48 teaspoons
1 cup = 1/2 pint
1 cup = 1/4 quart
1 cup = 1/16 gallon
1 cup = 240 ml.

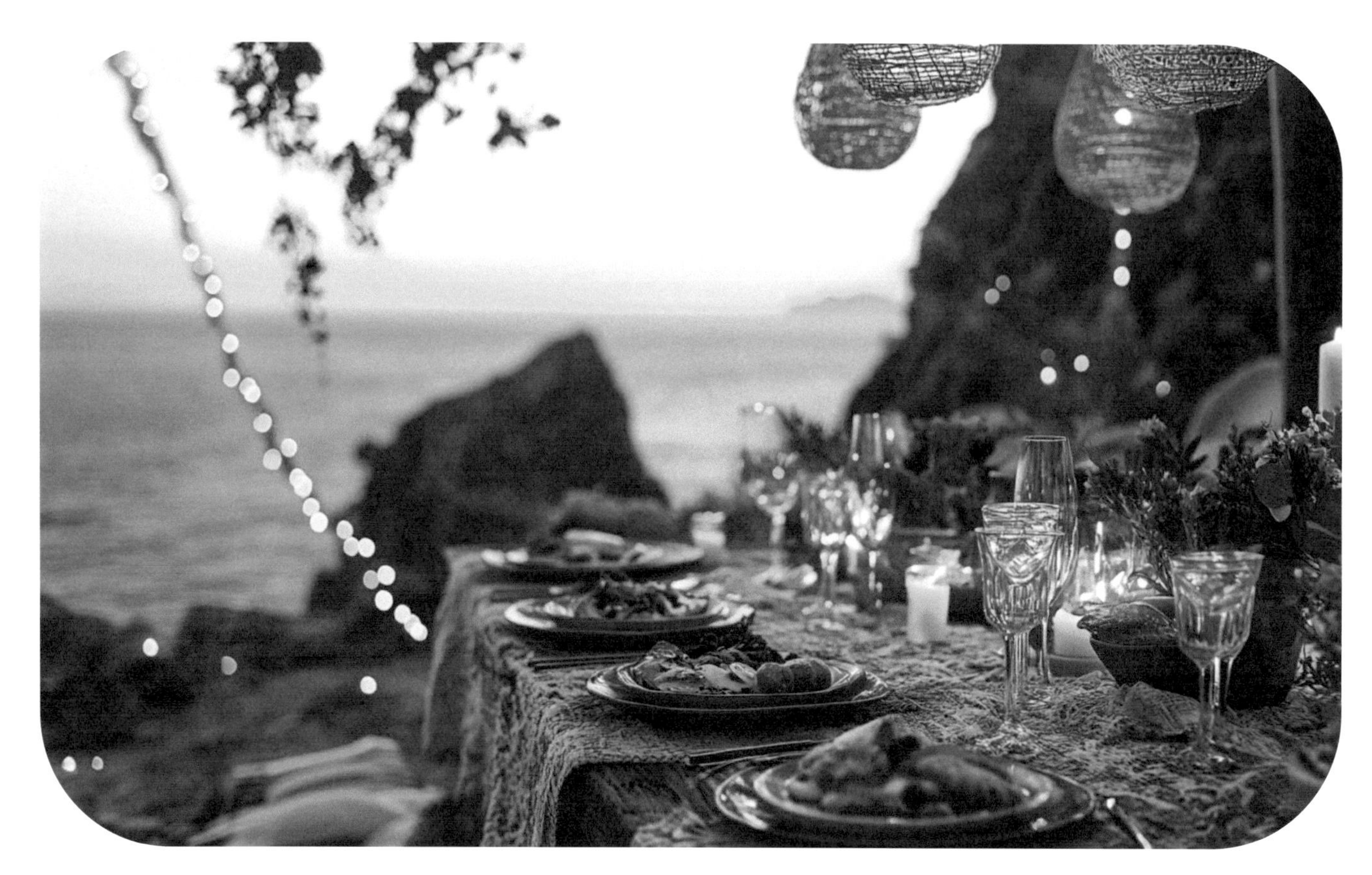

GRATITUDE

Dear Customer,

Thank you for choosing **"30-Minute Mediterranean Diet Cookbook for Beginners."** Your support means the world to me and my family. I'm truly grateful that you've welcomed this book into your kitchen. I hope these recipes inspire you to embrace the vibrant flavors, wholesome ingredients, and joyful spirit of Mediterranean cooking. Whether you're new to this lifestyle or looking to expand your culinary repertoire, I believe this book will help you create delicious, healthy meals that nourish both body and soul.

Cooking is more than just a daily task; it's an opportunity to connect with the people we love and the traditions we cherish. With this book, I hope to bring a bit of that warmth and connection into your home. I am honored that you've chosen to embark on this culinary journey with me, and I can't wait to hear about the memories you create around your table. Your trust in these recipes is a gift I don't take lightly, and I'm committed to making your cooking experience as enjoyable and rewarding as possible.

Thank you for being a part of this journey and for allowing me to be a part of yours.

With gratitude,

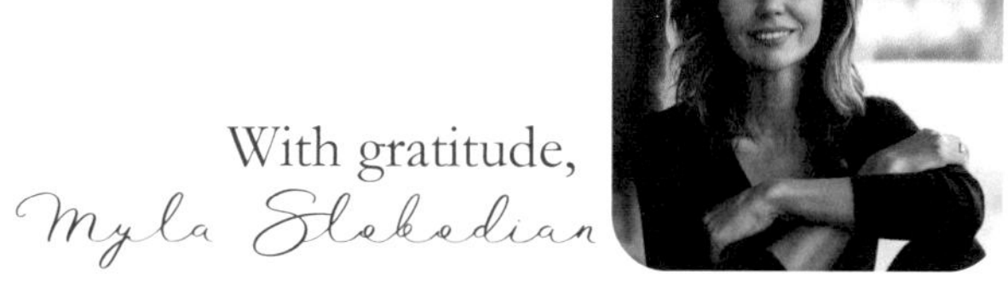

Made in the USA
Columbia, SC
29 December 2024

5baad6b8-42d7-4713-8bd1-b6addf49efbcR01